ATLAS OF
Oral and Maxillofacial Pathology

Joseph A. Regezi, DDS, MS

Professor, Oral Pathology
University of California
Divison of Oral Pathology
San Francisco, California

James J. Sciubba, DMD, PhD

Chairman, Department of Dental Medicine
Long Island Jewish Medical Center
New Hyde Park, New York

M. Anthony Pogrel, MB, ChB, BDS

Professor and Chairman
Department of Oral and Maxillofacial Surgery
University of California, San Francisco
San Francisco, California

W.B. Saunders Company
A Division of Harcourt Brace & Company
Philadelphia   London   Toronto   Montreal   Sydney   Tokyo

W.B. SAUNDERS COMPANY

A Division of Harcourt Brace & Company

The Curtis Center
Independence Square West
Philadelphia, Pennsylvania 19106

Library of Congress Cataloging-in-Publication Data
Regezi, Joseph A
        Atlas of oral and maxillofacial pathology / Joseph A. Regezi, M.
Anthony Pogrel, James J. Sciubba.—1st ed.
        p.   cm.
    ISBN 0–7216–8460–2
    1. Mouth—Disease Atlases.   2. Jaw—Diseases Atlases.
I. Pogrel, M. Anthony II. Sciubba, James J. III. Title.
    [DNLM: 1. Pathology, Oral Atlases.   2. Jaw Diseases, pathology
Atlases.   WU 17 R333a 2000]
RC815.R386 2000
617.5′207—dc21.
for Library of Congress   99–26383

NOTICE

Oral Pathology is an ever-changing field. Standard safety precautions must be followed, but as new research and clinical experience broaden our knowledge, changes in treatment and drug therapy become necessary or appropriate. Readers are advised to check the product information currently provided by the manufacturer of each drug to be administered to verify the recommended dose, the method and duration of administration, and the contraindications. It is the responsibility of the treatment physician, relying on experience and knowledge of the patient, to determine dosages and the best treatment for the patient. Neither the publisher nor the editor assumes any responsibility for any injury and/or damage to persons or property.

The Publisher

ATLAS OF ORAL AND MAXILLOFACIAL PATHOLOGY   ISBN–07216–8460–2

Preface

Atlas of Oral and Maxillofacial Pathology amalgamates the views and experiences of two oral and maxillofacial pathologists (JAR & JJS) and one oral and maxillofacial surgeon (MAP). We believe that our combined, and different, experiences in the diagnosis and treatment of oral diseases as reflected in this work make this atlas better than if it was authored by any one of us.

This color atlas is clinically oriented, but includes many representative photomicrographs that serve to link tissue changes with clinical appearances. We are convinced that these clinical-pathologic correlations are important in the understanding of oral disease processes. A comprehension of basic histopathology can proivde the clinician with a significant diagnostic advantage. It will also help in the interpretation of biopsy reports, and in the explanation of oral diseases to patients.

The all-color format and the chapter organizations are intended to assist the clinician in the development of clinical differential diagnoses. Clinicians preparing for board examinations should find the logical clinically oriented format helpful in reviewing the essential features of oral diseases. Our medical colleagues who may have the occasion to see patients with oral lesions/conditions should also find the illustrations and discussions helpful.

The material in the narrative portion of the atlas represents current thinking in oral and maxillofacial pathology, although it does not have the detail that one might occasionally need from a formal textbook, such as *Oral Pathology: Clinical Pathologic Correlation*, by Regezi and Sciubba (published by W.B. Saunders). The reader is referred to this or one of the other texts on the market for expansion of the conditions discussed and illustrated in the atlas.

Finally, we would like to acknowledge the work of W.B. Saunders Editor-in-Chief, Judith Fletcher, and her excellent professional staff, and Mary McDonald, P.M. Gordon Associates. We are grateful for their dedication to quality, and for their skills in bringing this work through the production and marketing processes.

Joseph A. Regezi
James J. Sciubba
M. Anthony Pogrel

Contents

ATLAS OF

Oral and Maxillofacial Pathology

Vesiculo-Bullous-Ulcerative Lesions

Neoplastic

Squamous Cell Carcinoma

Reactive

Traumatic Ulcer

Traumatic Granuloma

Necrotizing Sialometaplasia

Bacterial

Acute Necrotizing Ulcerative Gingivitis

Syphilis

Tuberculosis

Viral

Herpes Simplex Infections

Varicella and Herpes Zoster

Herpangina

Hand, Foot, and Mouth Disease

Fungal

Deep Fungal Infections

Mucormycosis and Aspergillosis

Immune Dysfunction

Drug Reactions and Angioedema

Aphthous Ulcers, Behçet's Syndrome, Reiter's Syndrome, and Crohn's Disease

Erythema Multiforme

Lupus Erythematosus

Pemphigus Vulgaris

Mucous Membrane Pemphigoid

Epidermolysis Bullosa

Midline Granuloma and Wegener's Granulomatosis

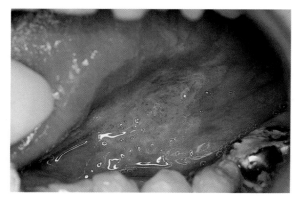

FIG. 1-1. Squamous cell carcinoma of lateral tongue

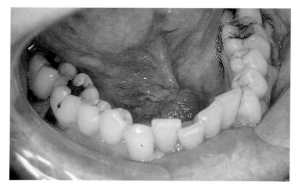

FIG. 1-2. Squamous cell carcinoma of floor of mouth

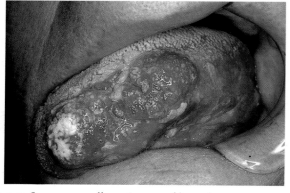

FIG. 1-3. Squamous cell carcinoma of lateral tongue

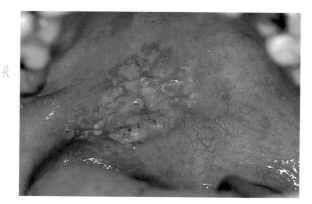

FIG. 1-4. Squamous cell carcinoma of palate

■ Squamous Cell Carcinoma

More than 90% of oral malignancies are squamous cell carcinomas. Annually in the United States, there are nearly 30,000 new cases and more than 9,000 deaths due to oral squamous cell carcinoma. In other parts of the world, such as India and Southeast Asia, where tobacco habits are much more intense, the relative incidence of oral cancer is much higher. For the past several decades, there has been only a slight improvement in the overall 5-year survival rate, from about 45% to 50%.

ETIOLOGY AND PATHOGENESIS

All forms of tobacco (including smokeless) are important causative agents of oral cancer. Human papilloma virus (subtypes 16 and 18) has been associated with some oral cancers, particularly verrucous forms. Alcohol and chronic irritation are regarded as modifying rather than initiating factors.

Etiologic factors are believed to be able to alter keratinocyte genes through mutation, amplification, and/or deletion, resulting in loss of control of cell cycle (increased proliferation and reduced apoptosis) and gain of cell motility. *p53*, a key negative regulator of the cell cycle, is mutated in many oral cancers. Several other cell cycle proteins may be over- or underexpressed, contributing to the process of malignant transformation. Some of these key cell cycle proteins that may be dysregulated in oral cancer and precancer are illustrated in Figure 1–5. Figure 1–6 is an immunohistochemical stain for presumably nonfunctional p53 protein in an oral cancer; the intensely positive nuclear staining signifies that p53 protein is dysregulated in this malignancy. Defective p53 allows cells to proceed into the S phase of the cell cycle before DNA can be repaired. The result is an accumulation of deleterious genetic defects that can lead to malignant transformation.

CLINICAL FEATURES

Oral cancer appears most commonly in the lateral tongue (25% to 40%) and the floor of the mouth (15% to 20%). It may appear as a nonhealing ulcer (Figs. 1–1 and 1–2), an irregular mass (Figs. 1–3 and 1–4), a red patch (erythroplakia), or a white patch (leukoplakia). In early stages it is painless. Metastasis, typically associated with a lesion greater than 2 cm in diameter, is usually to ipsilateral submandibular or jugulodigastric nodes.

MICROSCOPIC FEATURES

Most oral cancers are well to moderately differentiated (Figs. 1–7 through 1–10). Figure 1–12 shows the lymph node metastasis from the lesion illustrated in Figure 1–11; note the similar microscopic features in primary and secondary lesions. Cellular atypia, mitotic figures, and invasive patterns are highly variable. Diagnosis is based on nuclear detail and microscopic pattern. Microscopic variants include spindle cell carcinoma (sarcoma look-alike), basaloid-squamous (basal and squamous features), and verrucous carcinoma (see Chap. 4).

TREATMENT

Surgery and radiation continue to be the mainstays of oral cancer treatment. Clinical stage, much more than microscopic classification, determines which modality is used and when. Chemotherapy may be used in late-stage disease for palliation.

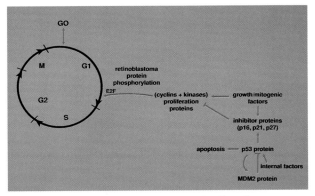

FIG. 1–5. Key G1–S proteins that control cell cycle

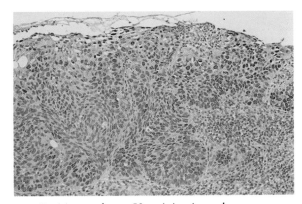

FIG. 1–6. Positive nuclear p53 staining in oral cancer

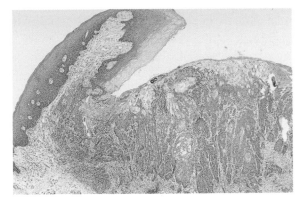

FIG. 1–7. Squamous cell carcinoma, lateral tongue

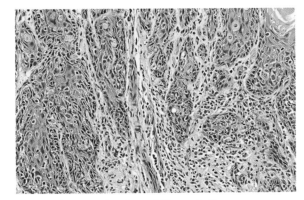

FIG. 1–8. High magnification of Figure 1–7

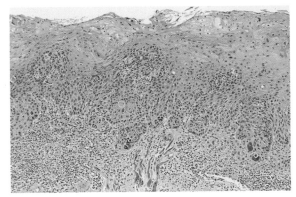

FIG. 1–9. Invasive squamous cell carcinoma, 29-year-old woman

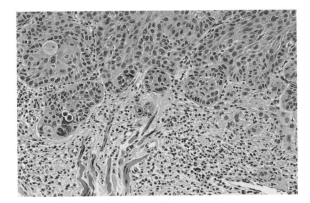

FIG. 1–10. High magnification of Figure 1–9

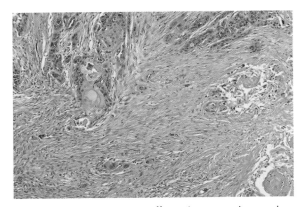

FIG. 1–11. Invasive squamous cell carcinoma, primary site

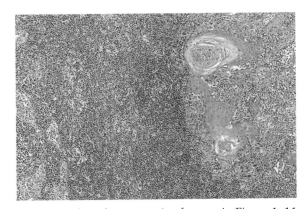

FIG. 1–12. Lymph node metastasis of tumor in Figure 1–11

CHAPTER 1: Vesiculo-Bullous-Ulcerative Lesions ■ *Neoplastic*

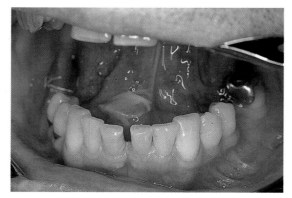

FIG. 1–13. Acute traumatic ulcer in floor of mouth

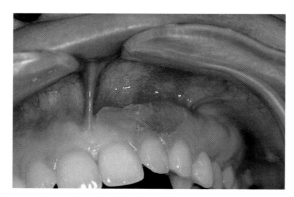

FIG. 1–14. Acute chemical-induced ulcer

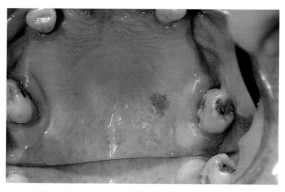

FIG. 1–15. Chronic traumatic ulcer of palate

■ Traumatic Ulcer

Ulcers are among the most common lesions seen in oral mucous membranes. Although there are many causes of oral ulcers, the unifying feature is simply loss of surface epithelium.

ETIOLOGY

Most of the ulcers seen in oral mucosa are a result of trauma. The cause of acute traumatic ulcers is usually apparent from patient history. The cause of chronic ulcers, however, may be less obvious because the injury may have been forgotten, or may be of very low grade.

Ulcers may be related to excessive heat or chemicals applied to mucosa, either by the dentist (iatrogenic injury) or by the patient. The oral mucosa is occasionally the site of factitial injury in patients with psychological problems.

CLINICAL FEATURES

Acute ulcers are painful. They usually have a yellow fibrinous base surrounded by an erythematous inflammatory halo (Figs. 1–13 and 1–14). Chronic ulcers, on the other hand, are associated with little or no pain. The ulcer base is generally yellow due to fibrin deposition or possibly red due to granulation tissue accumulation (Fig. 1–15). The margins of a chronic ulcer are usually elevated and firm due to scarring. Chronic ulcers mimic both chronic infectious ulcers and ulceration associated with mucosal malignancies. For reasons that are not well understood, chronic ulcers of the lateral border of the tongue frequently take a protracted length of time to heal. Another slow-to-heal ulcer is seen in the palate and is known as *necrotizing sialometaplasia*.

MICROSCOPIC FEATURES

Acute ulcers show loss of epithelium with fibrin covering the connective tissue base (Figs. 1–16 and 1–17). Neutrophils are seen within the fibrin membrane. Chronic ulcers also show infiltration by chronic inflammatory cells and evidence of repair. Scar is seen at the base of the lesion, and granulation tissue is found between the scar and the overlying precipitated fibrin. The inflammatory cell infiltrate is mixed. Epithelium at the ulcer margin may show evidence of regeneration in the form of epithelial cells between the fibrin membrane and subjacent viable granulation tissue. The so-called *traumatic granuloma* is a chronic ulcer in which there is a marked macrophage and eosinophil infiltrate.

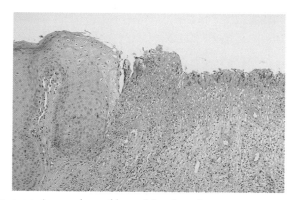

FIG. 1–16. Acute ulcer of lateral border of tongue

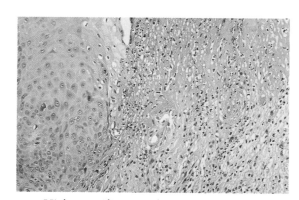

FIG. 1–17. High magnification of acute ulcer in Figure 1–16

CHAPTER 1: Vesiculo-Bullous-Ulcerative Lesions ■ *Reactive*

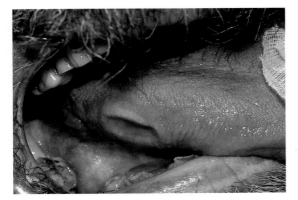

FIG. 1–18. Traumatic granuloma (chronic ulcer)

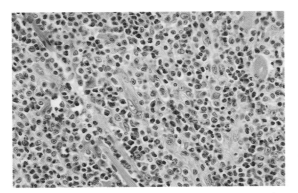

FIG. 1–19. Traumatic granuloma with macrophages and eosinophils

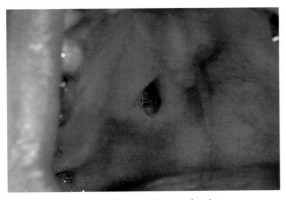

FIG. 1–20. Necrotizing sialometaplasia of palate

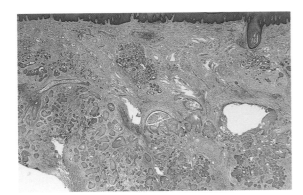

FIG. 1–21. Necrotizing sialometaplasia

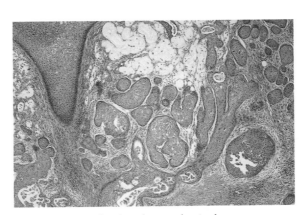

FIG. 1–22. Necrotic gland and metaplastic ducts

■ Traumatic Granuloma

Clinically, traumatic granuloma appears as a relatively painless crateriform ulcer with indurated margins (Fig. 1–18). The lateral tongue and occasionally the lip or buccal mucosa are affected. Delayed healing is typical. Biopsy is generally required to separate this lesion from squamous cell carcinoma and chronic infection.

This is a chronic ulcer in which there is an intense macrophage and eosinophil infiltrate (Fig. 1–19). Inflammation typically extends deep into subjacent muscle. The intense mononuclear infiltrate may suggest lymphoma or Langerhans cell disease.

■ Necrotizing Sialometaplasia

This chronic ulcer typically occurs in the hard palate in the region of the accessory salivary glands (Fig. 1–20). Ischemic necrosis of glandular tissue results in a sharply marginated ulcer. The condition is occasionally bilateral. Prolonged healing and pain are typical.

Microscopically, lobules of salivary gland show necrosis and ductal squamous metaplasia (Figs. 1–21 and 1–22). The lobular architecture of the glandular tissue persists, however. The center of the lesion is ulcerated. The combination of these features may suggest diagnoses such as squamous cell carcinoma and mucoepidermoid carcinoma.

Necrotizing sialometaplasia is a self-limiting process that does not require treatment other than biopsy to confirm the diagnosis. The lesion generally heals without sequelae.

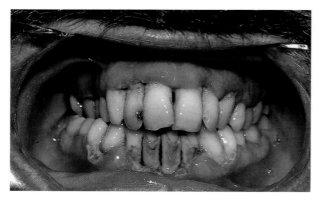
FIG. 1–23. Acute necrotizing ulcerative gingivitis

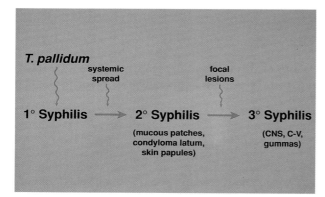
FIG. 1–24. Pathogenesis of syphilis

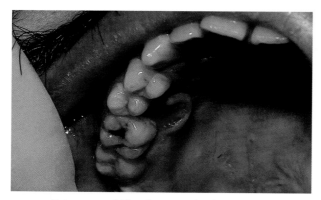
FIG. 1–25. Primary syphilis, chancre of palate

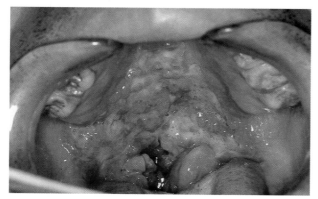
FIG. 1–26. Tertiary syphilis, palatal gumma

■ Acute Necrotizing Ulcerative Gingivitis

Also known as *Vincent's infection*, this is an opportunistic phenomenon in which oral fusiform bacteria and spirochetes proliferate in the gingiva of patients with predisposing conditions, including poor oral hygiene, poor nutrition, stress, smoking, and immunodeficiency. Seen most commonly in young adults, this form of gingivitis presents as generalized ulceration and necrosis of the marginal gingiva and interdental papillae (Fig. 1–23). The condition is painful, the patient has fetid breath, and bleeding may occur through the necrotic tissue. Treatment includes débridement and prophylaxis, improved oral hygiene, and occasionally antibiotics.

■ Syphilis

Syphilis is a sexually transmitted disease that may appear as oral ulceration(s) at any stage of the disease (Fig. 1–24). Syphilis can mimic both clinically and microscopically many of the chronic ulcerations listed in this chapter.

Syphilis is caused by direct sexual transmission of the spirochete *Treponema pallidum*. The lesion at the site of primary contact and infection is known as a chancre (Fig. 1–25). This lesion presents as a painless chronic ulcer and heals spontaneously after several weeks without treatment. After a latent period in which there is systemic dissemination of the microorganism, secondary syphilis develops in the form of a skin rash and oral ulcers with a mucoid exudate (mucous patch). Also seen are wartlike lesions known as condyloma latum. Patients who continue without treatment run the risk of developing tertiary lesions known as gummas (Fig. 1–26) and inflammatory lesions in the cardiovascular system and brain. The disease can be transmitted to a fetus by an infected mother. Numerous stigmata may result in the infected child, including Hutchinson's triad (misshapen first molars and incisors, ocular keratitis, eighth nerve deafness).

Clinically, the chancre appears as an indurated ulcer with rolled margins. The lesion is generally painless, but infectious. When occurring orally, most lesions appear on the lips, although any intraoral site may be affected. The lesion is often confused with carcinoma. Mucous patches may occur on any surface and are usually multiple and also infectious. The verruciform condyloma lata may occur on skin or mucosal surfaces. Gummas appear as necrotic destructive ulcers at any site. Palatal lesions may result in perforation to the nasal cavity.

Microscopically, the chronic inflammatory response to *T. pallidum* is generally nonspecific. However, plasma cells are usually seen in abundance and typically in a perivascular distribution. The ulcer itself has a nonspecific appearance. Silver stains may demonstrate the spirochete in tissue sections, especially from primary and secondary lesions.

Syphilis continues to be a public health problem and is increasing in incidence. Penicillin remains the drug of choice and continues to be effective in the treatment of most patients.

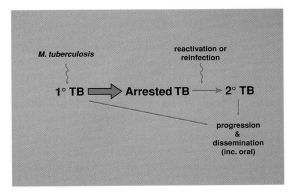

FIG. 1–27. Pathogenesis of tuberculosis

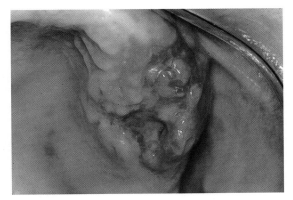

FIG. 1–28. Tuberculosis of alveolar ridge

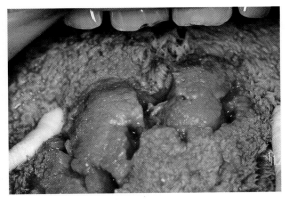

FIG. 1–29. Tuberculosis of tongue

■ Tuberculosis

Tuberculosis (TB) is a chronic disease predominantly of pulmonary tissue. Oral lesions are typically secondary to lung disease and appear as chronic nonhealing ulcers.

ETIOLOGY AND PATHOGENESIS

TB is caused by *Mycobacterium tuberculosis*. The increasing incidence of this disease has been related to urban living in which there are poor living conditions and compromised immunity. AIDS patients are at a significant risk for TB.

TB is spread through airborne droplets that carry organisms to lung tissue. This results in a primary infection that usually produces subclinical changes and arrested disease (Fig. 1–27). The organism can persist in a latent stage in the lung, and may be reactivated after compromise of the patient's systemic health. Oral TB usually follows reactivated or secondary TB.

CLINICAL FEATURES

Signs of clinical disease include fever, night sweats, malaise, and weight loss. Cough, hemoptysis, and chest pain signal pulmonary involvement. Microorganisms in infected sputum may become implanted in oral mucosa, resulting in indurated, chronic, nonhealing ulcer(s) (Figs. 1–28 and 1–29). Lesions may appear in any mucosal site, although the gingiva and tongue are frequently favored. Clinical differential diagnosis would generally include chronic traumatically induced ulcer and malignant neoplasm.

The treatment strategy of this disease has changed because of drug-resistant forms of TB. Multidrug therapeutic regimens include isoniazid, rifampin, streptomycin, and other drugs. Duration of therapy may extend into years.

MICROSCOPIC FEATURES

M. tuberculosis incites a chronic granulomatous reaction (Fig. 1–30). Focal areas of macrophages (granulomas) are surrounded by lymphocytes and fibroblasts. Fused macrophages result in giant cells of Langhans type (nuclei distributed around cell periphery). Central caseous necrosis is seen in the granulomas. The microorganism can be seen with special stains (Ziehl-Neelsen and Fite) in macrophages and giant cells (Fig. 1–31).

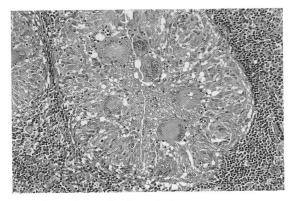

FIG. 1–30. Granuloma of tuberculosis

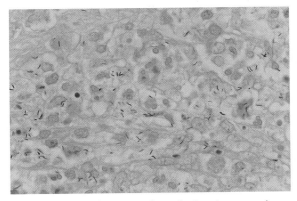

FIG. 1–31. Fite stain showing tuberculosis microorganisms

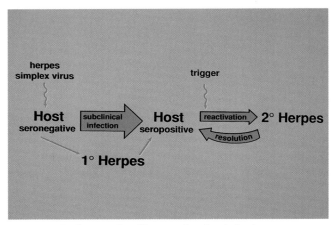

FIG. 1-32. Pathogenesis of herpes simplex infections

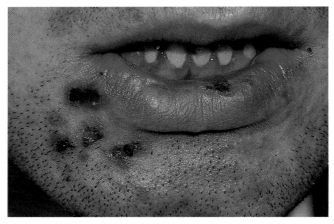

FIG. 1-33. Primary herpes simplex infection in an adult

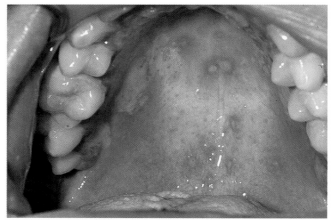

FIG. 1-34. Primary herpes simplex infection in an adult

■ Herpes Simplex Infections

Herpes simplex virus causes self-limited and potentially recurrent cutaneous and mucosal disease. In the primary form, most patients have subclinical disease, but a few develop systemic symptoms of viral infection and focal areas of vesicular eruption. In the secondary form, systemic signs are absent, but localized vesicular disease occurs.

ETIOLOGY AND PATHOGENESIS

Herpes simplex infections are transmitted through physical contact with an infected individual. After an incubation period of approximately 10 days, primary disease occurs but is usually subclinical (Fig. 1–32). A few patients develop overt disease in which there is vesicular eruption of the oral and perioral tissues along with headache, fever, and elevated temperature. After primary exposure, the virus may find its way to ganglion cells (e.g., trigeminal ganglion). Here the virus remains in a latent state and may be reactivated by sunlight, cold, trauma, stress, and immunosuppression. The virus travels by an unknown mechanism along the nerve to the site of the originally infected surface, such as the lips. Up to 90% of the population is seropositive for this virus. Less than half of this group develop secondary lesions.

CLINICAL FEATURES

Primary disease is typically seen in children as ulcers (from vesicles) and inflammation of the lips and gingiva in the context of systemic viral infection (Figs. 1–33 and 1–34). The self-limited course of 1 to 2 weeks can be shortened with the early introduction of oral acyclovir. Secondary or recurrent herpes infections usually affect the lips and surrounding skin (Figs. 1–35 and 1–36). Intraorally, it is almost always in the hard palate or gingiva (Figs. 1–37 and 1–38). Immunosuppressed patients may have lesions on any mucosal site. Lesions are preceded by prodromal symptoms of tingling and burning followed by multiple vesicles. The vesicles are short-lived and quickly break to become coalescent ulcers. Differential diagnosis for primary disease would include erythema multiforme and possibly acute necrotizing ulcerative gingivitis. Systemic symptoms as well as ulcers of the gingiva and palate are less likely in erythema multiforme. Secondary disease may be confused with aphthous ulcers, especially in HIV-positive patients. The different regional distribution for herpes and aphthous ulcers is generally a very helpful differentiating feature.

MICROSCOPIC FEATURES

Effects of this virus are found in the nuclei of keratinocytes. Lesions biopsied early during the course of this infection show characteristic nuclear changes (Figs. 1–39 and 1–40). Nuclei are smudgy, with chromatin peripherally distributed along the nuclear membrane. Multinucleated keratinocytes with these nuclear changes are also evident. Biopsy is usually unnecessary because diagnosis is possible from clinical features. Recurrent disease in AIDS and transplant patients will likely show atypical distribution, making biopsy or cytology desirable.

Cure is difficult to achieve in patients with herpes simplex infection. Control can be accomplished with oral acyclovir. Acyclovir may be used as a prophylactic agent to prevent severe secondary herpes seen in association with immunosuppression.

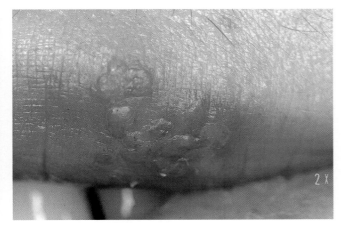

FIG. 1–35. Secondary herpes simplex infection of lip

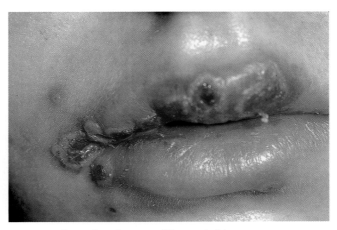

FIG. 1–36. Secondary herpes of lips and skin

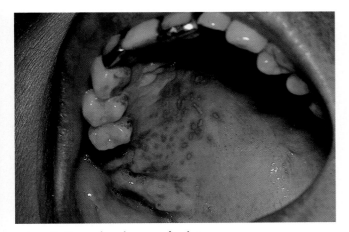

FIG. 1–37. Secondary herpes of palate

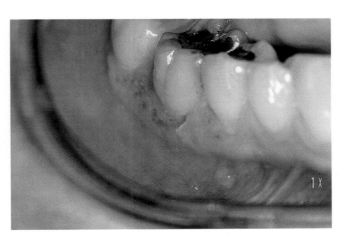

FIG. 1–38. Secondary herpes of gingiva

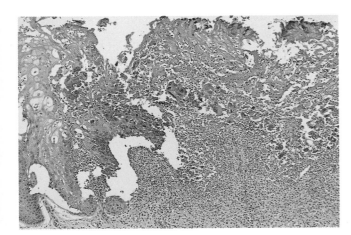

FIG. 1–39. Ulcer of secondary herpes

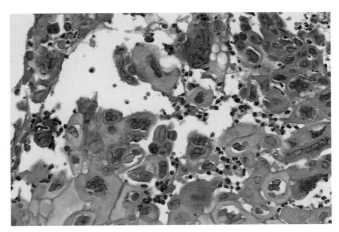

FIG. 1–40. Keratinocytes with nuclear herpes virus inclusions

CHAPTER 1: Vesiculo-Bullous-Ulcerative Lesions ■ *Viral*

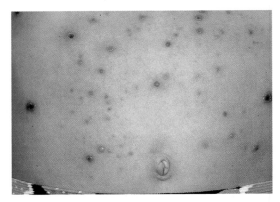

FIG. 1–41. Vesiculobullous eruption of varicella

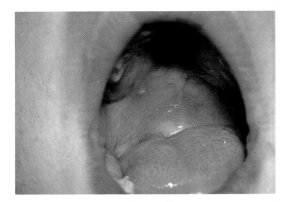

FIG. 1–42. Oral expression of varicella

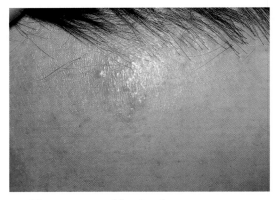

FIG. 1–43. Herpes zoster of forehead

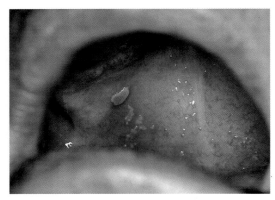

FIG. 1–44. Intraoral herpes zoster

■ Varicella

Varicella zoster virus is responsible for primary disease, varicella (*chickenpox*), and secondary disease, herpes zoster (*shingles*). This is a herpes virus that causes muco-cutaneous disease, similar in many ways to herpes simplex infections. Skin eruptions dominate the clinical picture, and oral manifestations are infrequent.

PATHOGENESIS
Varicella is predominantly a childhood viral infection that is transmitted through contaminated droplets and less often by direct contact. After a 10-day incubation period, waves of vesicles appear on the skin. The viremia also elicits signs and symptoms of infection. The disease is self-limited (2 to 3 weeks), with potential sequestration of virus in the sensory ganglia.

Herpes zoster may occur due to reactivation of latent virus, particularly in patients who are immunosuppressed. This would include patients who develop malignancies (e.g., lymphoma) and patients who receive drugs or radiation for malignancies. Zoster is the localized form of the disease and appears with intense pain or paresthesia that may persist well beyond the clinical healing phase.

CLINICAL FEATURES
The vesicular eruption associated with primary disease affects the trunk and head and neck areas predominantly (Fig. 1–41). The vesicles become pustular and ulcerate. Infrequently, oral mucosal lesions present as small shallow ulcers (Fig. 1–42). When occurring in adults and immuno-compromised patients, the disease may have a more severe clinical course.

■ Herpes Zoster

Herpes zoster presents as a vesicular eruption (Fig. 1–43), usually along the distribution of a sensory nerve of the trunk. The unilaterality of the eruption is characteristic; this unilaterality is evident in the oral lesions as well. Oral lesions appear as multiple, shallow ulcers preceded by short-lived vesicles (Fig. 1–44). Bone necrosis has also been described.

MICROSCOPIC FEATURES
Varicella zoster virus produces keratinocyte nuclear changes similar to those of herpes simplex virus infection. Smudgy gray nuclei with marginated chromatin indicate accumulation of virus and viral products.

TREATMENT
High-dose oral acyclovir (generally double the dose for herpes simplex infections) can help control this disease. Analgesics are generally required to reduce postherpetic pain.

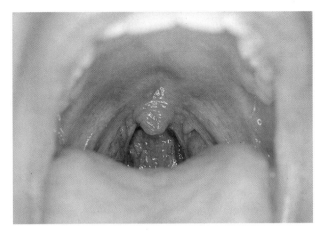

FIG. 1–45. Herpangina

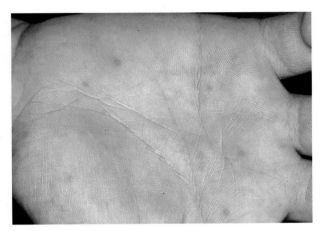

FIG. 1–46. Hand, foot, and mouth disease

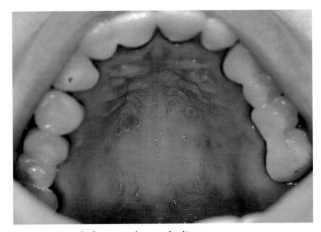

FIG. 1–47. Hand, foot, and mouth disease

■ Herpangina

Herpangina is an acute systemic viral infection. It is endemic and often seasonal (summer or fall). It is caused by one of several subtypes of coxsackie virus.

Clinically, children are usually affected and have signs and symptoms of acute viremia. There is also a vesicular-ulcerative eruption in the posterior part of the mouth. The soft palate, faucial pillars, and tonsils are usually affected, showing multiple ulcers (Fig. 1–45). The disease is mild to moderate in intensity, is self-limited, and provides lasting immunity.

Because of its self-limited and usually mild to moderate nature, treatment is supportive. Complications are rare.

■ Hand, Foot, and Mouth Disease

This is an acute viral infection caused by members of the coxsackievirus group. The several subtypes that may cause this disease are different from those that cause herpangina. The disease is endemic and self-limited.

Clinically, after a short incubation period of 1 week, signs and symptoms of systemic viral infection (fever, malaise, lymphadenopathy) appear in conjunction with small vesiculo-ulcerative lesions of the mucous membranes, feet, and hands (Figs. 1–46 and 1–47). Lesions heal uneventfully without scar.

There is no virus-specific therapy for hand, foot, and mouth disease. Management is symptomatic.

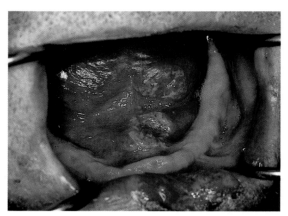

FIG. 1–48. Histoplasmosis of oral floor and lip

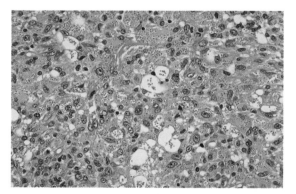

FIG. 1–49. Macrophages containing *Histoplasma capsulatum*

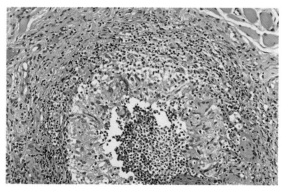

FIG. 1–50. Blastomycosis—granuloma with central abscess

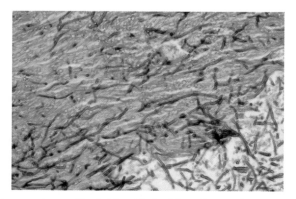

FIG. 1–51. Aspergillosis identified with a silver stain

■ Deep Fungal Infections

Deep fungal diseases usually present intraorally after organism implantation from primary pulmonary lesions. This group of diseases includes *histoplasmosis, coccidioidomycosis, blastomycosis,* and *cryptococcosis.*

The cause of pulmonary disease is believed to be related to inhalation of fungal spores. As lung disease advances, microorganisms are found in sputum, the presumed source of infection for mucous membranes. Histoplasmosis (*Histoplasma capsulatum*) and cryptococcosis (*Cryptococcus neoformans*) are endemic to the Midwestern United States. Coccidioidomycosis (*Coccidioides immitis*) is endemic to the West. Blastomycosis (*Blastomyces dermatitidis*) has a North American distribution.

Clinically, oral infection by the deep fungal organisms results in nonhealing, usually multiple, chronic ulcers (Fig. 1–48). These lesions may or may not occur concomitantly with systemic signs and symptoms of cough, fever, night sweats, weight loss, chest pain, and hemoptysis. Antifungal therapy includes amphotericin B, as well as other drugs such as ketoconazole and fluconazole.

Microscopically, deep fungi incite a granulomatous inflammatory response (Figs. 1–49 and 1–50). Macrophages and multinucleated giant cells are usually seen without necrosis. The size of the microorganisms usually allows visualization at high magnification (×400). Silver stains can be used to enhance these microorganisms.

■ Mucormycosis and Aspergillosis

These and other related fungal diseases are opportunistic in their behavior. Their overgrowth in human tissue is usually related to immunosuppression or debilitation.

The opportunistic mycotic microorganisms are ubiquitous in nature and are found in decaying food. The route of infection is believed to be either through the gastrointestinal or respiratory tract. A pre-existing systemic condition, such as uncontrolled diabetes, transplant recipient, advanced malignancy, or AIDS, typically precedes the overgrowth of these fungi.

Clinically, necrosis of the palate sinuses, and/or nasal tissues is the characteristic presentation of this condition. The lesions tend to be destructive and may perforate the palate. Differential diagnosis would include midline granuloma, Wegener's granulomatosis, tertiary syphilis, and malignant disease.

Microscopically, large branching fungi are seen in a nonspecific acute and chronic inflammatory cell infiltrate (Fig. 1–51). Necrosis, including blood vessel walls, is also present.

Amphotericin B is used to treat opportunistic fungal infections. Débridement may be required because of a fungal mass within a body cavity. Prognosis is dependent on the control of the patient's underlying condition.

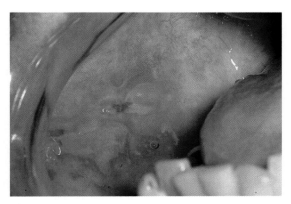

FIG. 1–52. Systemic drug-induced ulceration of the buccal mucosa

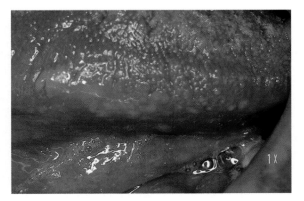

FIG. 1–53. Ulcers due to contact allergy to dental acrylic

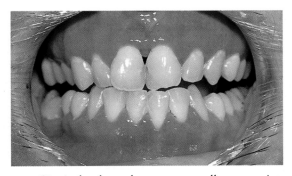

FIG. 1–54. Gingival redness due to contact allergy to mint

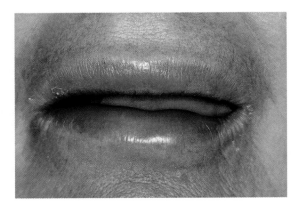

FIG. 1–55. Angioedema of lips

■ Drug Reactions and Angioedema

Mucosal reactions to systemic or topical drugs are highly variable and cannot be diagnosed from clinical appearance. Duration of drug, dosage, drug structure, and individual intrinsic responses are responsible for the variety of presenting appearances.

ETIOLOGY AND PATHOGENESIS

Untoward mucosal reactions to drugs may be related to immunologic or nonimmunologic responses. One of several mechanisms (humoral, cell-mediated, both) may be involved in hyperimmune responses. Nonimmunologic mechanisms, such as direct toxicity, do not stimulate the immune system and are not antibody-dependent. Contact allergy reactions are mediated by Langerhans cells. These dendritic cells, which are found in the epithelial prickle cell zone, process and present antigenic determinants to lymphocytes. Antigenic rechallenge to the same focus results in lymphocytic release of the chemical mediators of inflammation, resulting in clinical disease.

CLINICAL FEATURES

Mucosal lesions resulting from systemic drugs (Fig. 1–52) or topical allergens (Figs. 1–53 and 1–54) may exhibit a wide range of appearances, including swelling, redness, keratosis, ulceration, and vesiculation. The true incidence of mucosal reactions is unknown, and clinical diagnosis is often difficult. Correlation with a drug history is critical.

A distinctive form of drug reaction, known as *angioedema*, is IgE-mediated and is precipitated by drugs or food (especially nuts and shellfish). The condition progresses rapidly to produce soft, painless swelling of the lips, neck, and/or face (Fig. 1–55). There is no redness associated with the swelling. Most cases of this phenomenon are acquired, although there is a rare hereditary form in which patients have deficient or inadequate C1 esterase inhibitor (first component of complement).

MICROSCOPIC FEATURES

Although the histology of drug reactions is relatively nonspecific, some features that are usually seen include spongiosis, apoptotic basal keratinocytes, lymphoid infiltrates, and eosinophils. Reactions may be focused at the epithelial–connective tissue interface, mimicking lichen planus.

TREATMENT

Identification and removal of the offending drug or substance from the patient's regimen is essential. Antihistamines and corticosteroids may have some usefulness in disease management as well. This is particularly the case for angioedema.

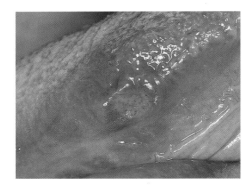

FIG. 1-56. Minor aphthous ulcer of tongue

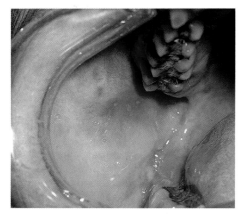

FIG. 1-57. Minor aphthous ulcers of buccal mucosa

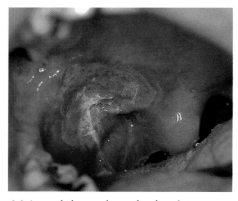

FIG. 1-58. Major aphthous ulcer of soft palate

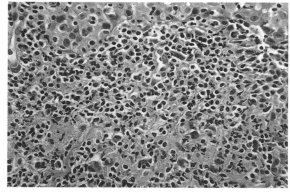

FIG. 1-59. Lymphocytes in preulcer stage (epithelium at top)

■ Aphthous Ulcers, Behçet's Syndrome, Reiter's Syndrome, and Crohn's Disease

Aphthous ulcers are recurrent painful mucosal lesions of unknown cause. They are self-limiting and can be controlled but not cured. Morbidity runs the spectrum of mild inconvenience to moderate debilitation.

Although the cause of aphthous ulcers is unknown, it is believed that they are related to a focal immune defect in which T lymphocytes play an early role. A viral cause has long been suspected but has not been substantiated. A small subset of aphthous ulcer patients appear to be deficient in vitamin B_{12}, folic acid, and/or iron. Hormonal alterations, stress, trauma, and food sensitivity are secondary or triggering factors. AIDS patients develop aphthous-like ulcers that are more severe.

Clinically, aphthous ulcers are classified into minor, major, and herpetiform types. The common minor type represents a relatively mild form of the disease. Minor aphthae are usually single, oval, and covered by fibrin surrounded by an erythematous halo (Figs. 1–56 and 1–57). The lesion is less than 0.5 cm. Prodromal symptoms of tingling and burning often precede ulceration. There is no vesicular stage. Only movable mucosa is affected; the dry vermilion is unaffected. Except in AIDS patients, the palate and hard gingiva are rarely affected. Major aphthous ulcers represent a larger, more severe form of aphthae (Fig. 1–58). These lesions range from 0.5 to 2 cm. They are crateriform and heal with scar. Several may be present at one time, and they may take several weeks to heal. Herpetiform (herpes-like) aphthae are multiple, usually seen in crops. They are not as site-restricted as minor and major lesions.

Microscopically, once ulceration has occurred, aphthous ulcers exhibit a nonspecific appearance. Before ulceration, an intense T-lymphocytic infiltrate is seen at the epithelial–connective tissue interface (Fig. 1–59). The triggering event is unknown. Rarely, cytomegalovirus may be seen in the base of these lesions; the significance of this finding is unknown.

The only reliable therapy with a scientific basis is topical or systemic corticosteroids. Generally, patients with minor aphthae request no treatment. Ulcers in more severely affected patients can be controlled with potent topical corticosteroids. Patients with intense disease may require short-term low- to intermediate-dose prednisone.

Behçet's syndrome is a multisystem disease that may affect not only the GI tract but also the cardiovascular system, eyes, CNS, joints, lung, and skin. Typically, mucous membrane ulceration is seen in the mouth (Fig. 1–60), eye (Fig. 1–61), and genitals. This is a serious disease in which vasculitis may play a role.

Reiter's syndrome is another mucocutaneous phenomenon of unknown cause. Major components include aphthous-like ulcers (Fig. 1–62), arthritis, urethritis, and conjunctivitis or uveitis.

Crohn's disease or regional ileitis, due to granulomatous inflammation of the ileum, may also produce manifestations in oral mucosa. These include aphthous-like ulcers (Fig. 1–63) and mucosal nodules with underlying granulomas (Figs. 1–64 and 1–65).

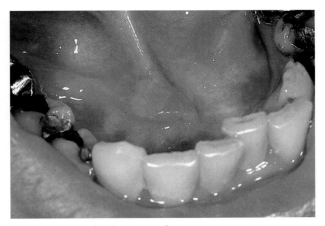

FIG. 1–60. Ulcer of Behçet's syndrome

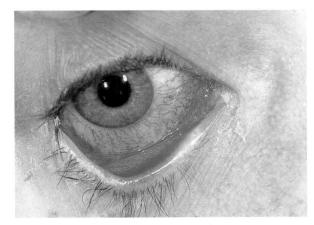

FIG. 1–61. Conjunctivitis of Behçet's syndrome

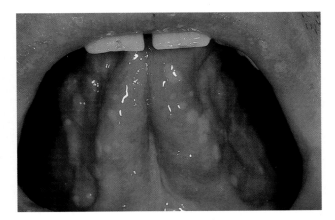

FIG. 1–62. Ulcers as part of Reiter's syndrome

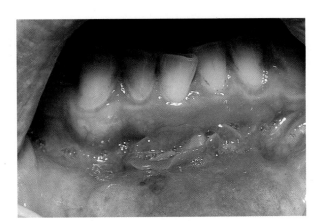

FIG. 1–63. Ulcers and fissures of Crohn's disease

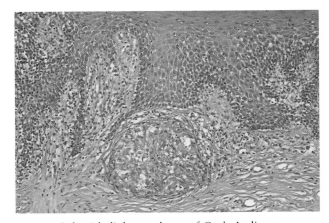

FIG. 1–64. Subepithelial granuloma of Crohn's disease

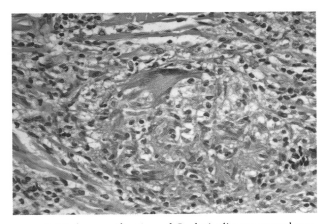

FIG. 1–65. High magnification of Crohn's disease granuloma

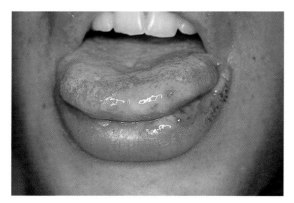

FIG. 1–66. Erythema multiforme ulcers of episode 1

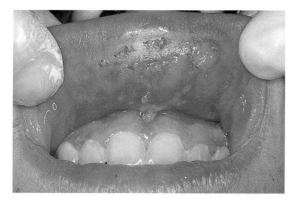

FIG. 1–67. Erythema multiforme ulcers of episode 2

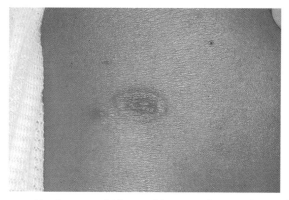

FIG. 1–68. Erythema multiforme skin target lesion of episode 2

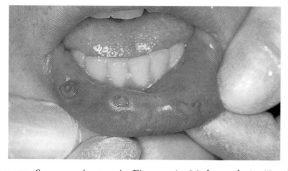

FIG. 1–69. Same patient as in Figures 1–66 through 1–68 with lip ulcers in episode 3

■ Erythema Multiforme

Erythema multiforme (EM) is an acute self-limited disease that is expressed in skin and/or mucous membranes. A wide spectrum of disease intensity has been observed, with mild cases referred to as EM minor and severe cases as EM major. When lesions are particularly severe and involve more than one mucosal site, the term *Stevens-Johnson syndrome* has been used. This term is often used synonymously with EM major.

ETIOLOGY
Generally, EM is believed to represent a hypersensitivity reaction. Most cases of EM minor are associated with a preceding herpes simplex virus episode. A hypersensitivity reaction to a viral antigen triggers the eruption. EM major has been associated, in part, with infections such as herpes simplex and mycoplasma, but also with drugs. Sulfa drugs have been the most frequently cited trigger of the major form of this disease.

CLINICAL FEATURES
The disease often appears suddenly as a cutaneous erythematous maculopapular rash. Some of the lesions may show concentric alternating red and white circles, described as target or iris lesions. When oral mucosal lesions are present, they appear as large, superficial ulcers of several regions of the mouth (Fig. 1–66). The gingiva is typically spared, a sign that helps differentiate this disease from primary herpes simplex infections. Systemic signs and symptoms are typically absent. Recurrence may be seen (Figs. 1–67 through 1–69), usually after an episode of recurrent herpes simplex infection.

Lesions of EM major are considerably more severe and may include inflammation of the conjunctiva (Figs. 1–70 and 1–71). Fever, malaise, and other clinical signs and symptoms may be associated with this form of the disease.

MICROSCOPIC FEATURES
Oral lesions initially show spongiosis in acanthotic epithelium (Figs. 1–72). Basal and parabasal keratinocytes show apoptotic change. Vesicles appear either at the epithelial–connective tissue interface or within the epithelium itself. Macrophages and lymphocytes dominate the inflammatory cell infiltrate. Large numbers of inflammatory cells are found at the epithelial–connective tissue interface, as well as in perivascular spaces of the deeper submucosa (Figs. 1–73 through 1–75).

TREATMENT
This disease is self-limited and typically requires only symptomatic support. In the major form of the disease, corticosteroids have been used, but significant beneficial effects have not been consistently achieved. For patients with recurrent herpes-triggered disease, prophylactic low dose acyclovir may help control rates of recurrence.

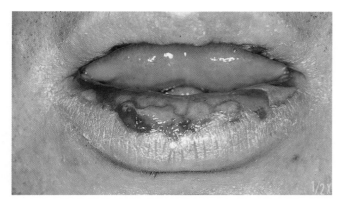

FIG. 1–70. EM major

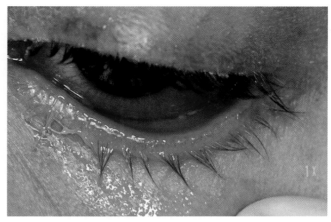

FIG. 1–71. Ocular lesions of patient in Figure 1–70

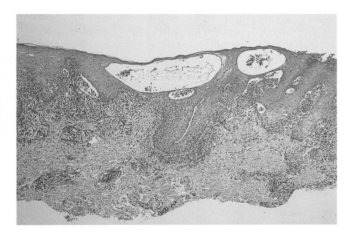

FIG. 1–72. Epithelial edema and lymphoid infiltrate in EM

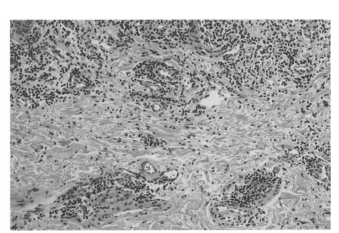

FIG. 1–73. Perivascular infiltrate in patient in Figure 1–72

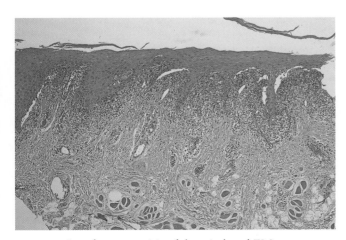

FIG. 1–74. Interface mucositis of drug-induced EM

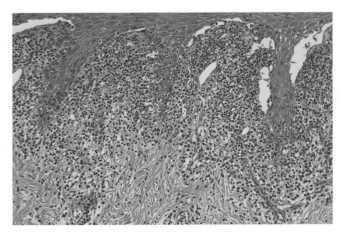

FIG. 1–75. High magnification of Figure 1–74

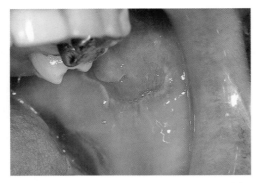

FIG. 1–76. Systemic lupus erythematosus—lichenoid lesion

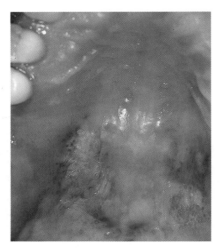

FIG. 1–77. Systemic lupus erythematosus with palatal lesions

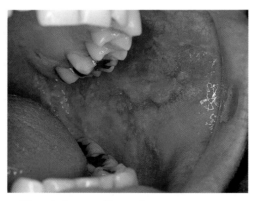

FIG. 1–78. Chronic lupus of buccal mucosa

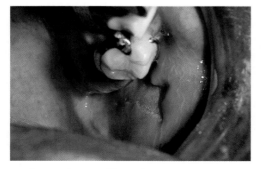

FIG. 1–79. Chronic lupus of buccal mucosa

■ Lupus Erythematosus

Lupus erythematosus is an autoimmune phenomenon that occurs in two well-recognized forms: systemic or acute, and chronic or discoid. Systemic lupus is a serious and potentially life-threatening disease that affects mucocutaneous tissues in addition to other organs such as the heart, kidney, and joints. Chronic or discoid lupus affects only the skin and/or mouth. Rarely does the chronic form develop into the systemic form.

ETIOLOGY

The trigger for this autoimmune process is unknown, although genetic and viral factors may play a role. Circulating autoantibodies to cytoplasmic and nuclear proteins are demonstrable in the systemic but not the chronic discoid form of the disease. T lymphocytes are also activated in this disease.

CLINICAL FEATURES

This disease results in erythematous lesions of the skin and mucous membranes. The lesions in the discoid form are generally more severe in these sites than the systemic form (Figs. 1–76 through 1–84). On the skin, erythematous patches expand peripherally and show central zones of scarring and hypopigmentation. Oral lesions are erythematous, often with central ulceration. Delicate punctate and striated white changes representing keratosis are seen around the periphery of the lesions.

MICROSCOPIC FEATURES

Characteristic features include epithelial atrophy, hyperkeratosis, and a lymphocytic infiltrate at the epithelial–connective tissue interface and in deep perivascular spaces (Figs 1–85 and 1–86). Microscopic differential diagnosis usually includes lichen planus and hypersensitivity reaction.

TREATMENT

The therapeutic goal is disease control. Corticosteroids, both topical and systemic, are recommended. Other immunosuppressive drugs may be used in difficult cases. Antimalarial agents are also often effective in this disease.

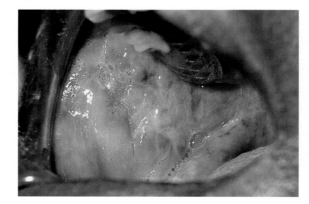

FIG. 1–80. Same patient as in Figure 1–79

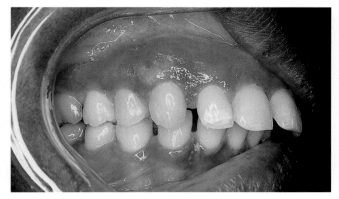
FIG. 1–81. Chronic lupus erythematosus of gingiva

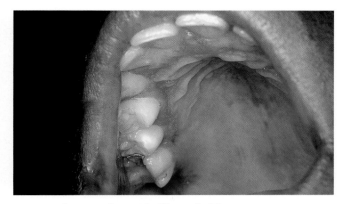
FIG. 1–82 Same patient as in Figure 1–81

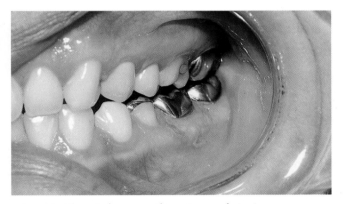
FIG. 1–83. Chronic lupus erythematosus of gingiva

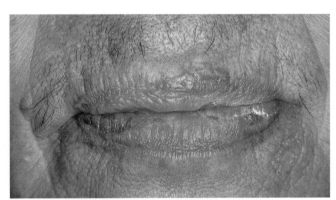
FIG. 1–84. Chronic lupus erythematosus of lips

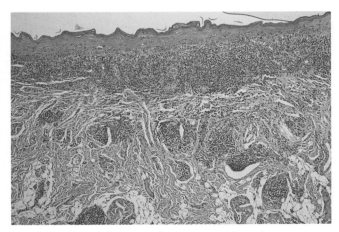
FIG. 1–85. Chronic lupus erythematosus of buccal mucosa

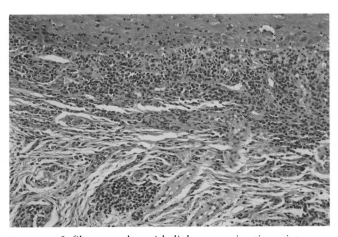
FIG. 1–86. Infiltrate at the epithelial–connective tissue interface

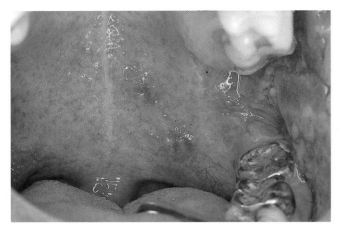

FIG. 1–87. Pemphigus bullae (palate) and ulcer (buccal mucosa)

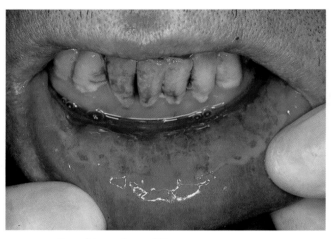

FIG. 1–88. Pemphigus ulcer of lip

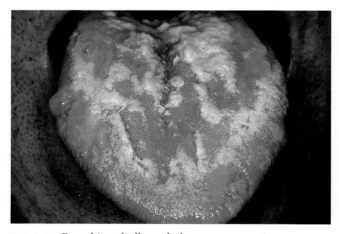

FIG. 1–89. Pemphigus bulla and ulcers on tongue (same patient in Figs. 1–87 through 1–89)

■ Pemphigus Vulgaris

This is an autoimmune mucocutaneous disease that results in multiple ulcers that are preceded by short-lived blisters. The lesions may be associated with painful debilitation, fluid loss, and electrolyte imbalance, making this a serious disease with potentially profound sequelae.

ETIOLOGY AND PATHOGENESIS
The triggering event of this autoimmune process is unknown. Circulating autoantibodies (IgG) are directed against an epithelial desmosomal protein known as desmoglein 3. The effect of the autoantibody–antigen reaction is the weakening of desmosomes and loss of cell-to-cell adhesion.

CLINICAL FEATURES
Oral lesions precede skin lesions in at least half of the patients. In both the skin and mucous membrane, lesions appear as ulcers (Fig. 1–96). The ulcers are preceded by short-lived bullae. Orally, lesions affect more than one mucosal region and are usually large and shallow (Figs. 1–87 through 1–89). Wearing of dental appliances may become difficult because of the production of new blisters associated with the rubbing of the appliances on the mucosa (Fig. 1–90). In some cases, lesions resemble aphthous ulcers (Figs. 1–91 and 1–92).

MICROSCOPIC FEATURES
The essential microscopic changes are intraepithelial separation with free-floating or acantholytic keratinocytes (Tzanck cells) (Figs. 1–93 and 1–94). Direct immunofluorescent examination of normal-appearing tissue adjacent to lesions exhibits a network of fluorescence representing the autoantibody–antigen complexes in the keratinocyte desmosomes (Fig. 1–95).

TREATMENT
Prednisone is the drug of choice for control of this disease. Because of their steroid-sparing effects, immunosuppressive agents such as azathioprine, methotrexate, and cyclophosphamide are often included in difficult cases.

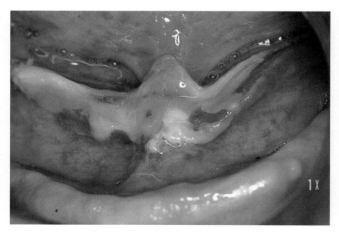

FIG. 1–90. Pemphigus in oral floor—denture-related

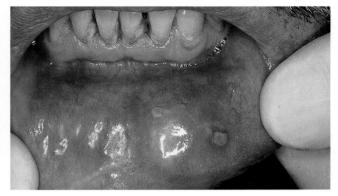

FIG. 1–91. Pemphigus vulgaris mimicking aphthous ulcers

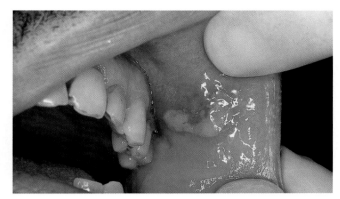

FIG. 1–92. Same patient as in Figure 1–91

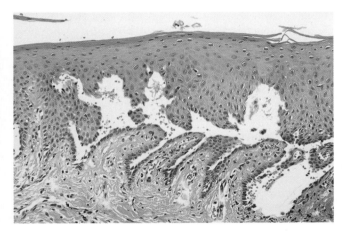

FIG. 1–93. Intraepithelial separation of pemphigus vulgaris

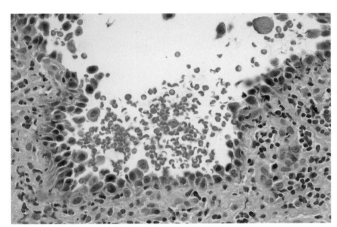

FIG. 1–94. Free-floating Tzanck cells in intraepithelial bulla

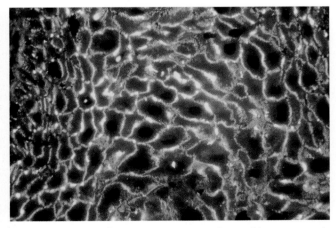

FIG. 1–95. Immunofluorescent staining of pemphigus autoantibodies

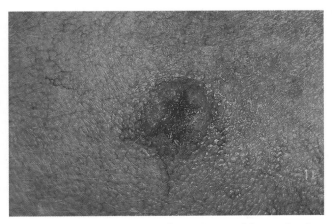

FIG. 1–96. Ulcerative cutaneous lesion in pemphigus vulgaris

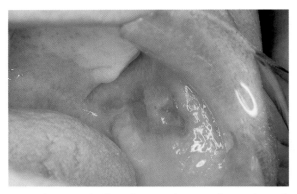

FIG. 1–97. Ulcerative-bullous lesion of mucosal pemphigoid

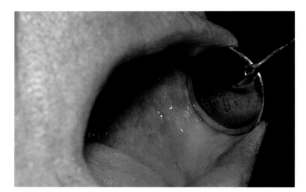

FIG. 1–98. Mucous membrane pemphigoid ulcer

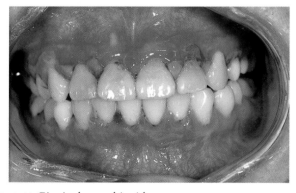

FIG. 1–99 Gingival pemphigoid

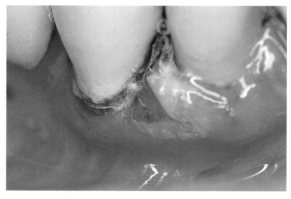

FIG. 1–100. Gingival pemphigoid showing epithelial separation

■ Mucous Membrane Pemphigoid

Mucous membrane pemphigoid, also known as *cicatricial pemphigoid*, is an autoimmune mucosal disease that infrequently affects the skin. Oral lesions are a source of chronic discomfort, and ocular lesions are potentially very serious because of conjunctival inflammation and scarring.

ETIOLOGY
How this disease is triggered is unknown. The autoantibodies that are produced are directed against basement membrane antigens, laminin 5, and so-called bullous pemphigoid antigen 230.

CLINICAL FEATURES
This is a disease of older adults (>50 years) and especially women. Patients present with patchy ulcers preceded by blisters. Although any area of the mucosa may be affected (Figs. 1–97 and 1–98, many patients have only gingival disease (Figs. 1–99 through 1–102). With chronicity, lesions may resemble lupus, lichen planus, and contact hypersensitivity. The lesions are persistent, although patients will have periods of improvement. Pain associated with the ulcerations decreases in intensity with time. A positive Nikolsky sign may be seen.

Conjunctival lesions may result in corneal damage in the form of scarring that can lead to blindness. Symblepharon is a complication of ocular pemphigoid (Fig. 1–106). Less commonly, lesions may be seen in the larynx, genitals, esophagus, and skin.

HISTOLOGIC FEATURES
Subepithelial separation is characteristic of this disease (Figs. 1–103 and 1–104). The pathologic space appears through the basement membrane, leaving basal keratinocytes intact in the epithelial roof of the bulla. Direct immunofluorescence shows linear deposits of IgG and C3 in the basement membrane zone (Fig. 1–105).

TREATMENT
Corticosteroids can be used to help control this disease. The addition of steroid-sparing immunosuppressive drugs may be required when ocular pemphigoid is present. For patients with chronic gingival disease, excellent oral hygiene with chlorhexidine rinses is of significant benefit in minimizing secondary inflammation. Some cases of gingival pemphigoid are refractory to low or intermediate doses of prednisone. Effective control of many of these cases can be achieved through the use of high-potency topical corticosteroids; high-dose prednisone is probably not warranted for this limited form of the disease.

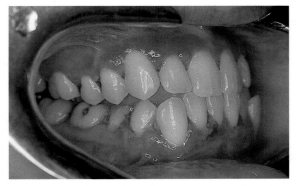

FIG. 1–101. Gingival pemphigoid presenting as red patches and ulcers

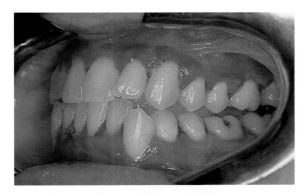

FIG. 1–102. Same patient as in Figure 1–100

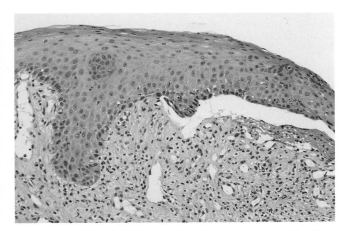

FIG. 1–103. Subepithelial separation in mucosal pemphigoid

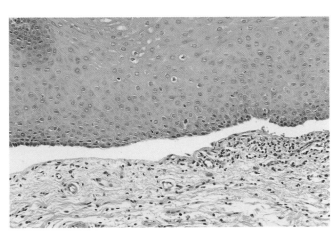

FIG. 1–104. Intact basal keratinocytes in pemphigoid bulla

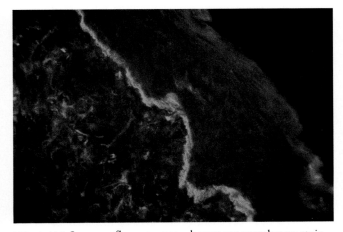

FIG. 1–105. Immunofluorescence—basement membrane stain

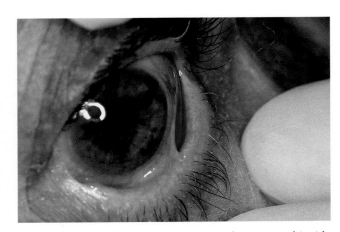

FIG. 1–106. Symblepharon in mucous membrane pemphigoid

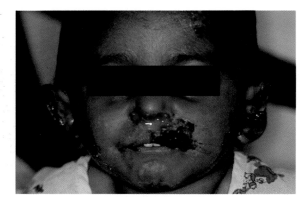

FIG. 1–107. Ulcers in epidermolysis bullosa

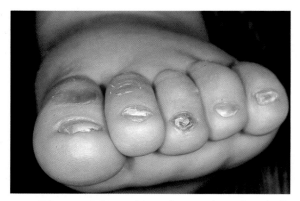

FIG. 1–108. Ulcers and dystrophic nails in epidermolysis bullosa

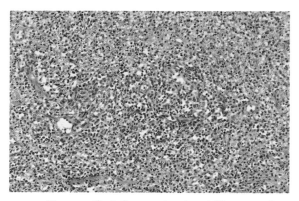

FIG. 1–109. Nonspecific inflammation in midline granuloma

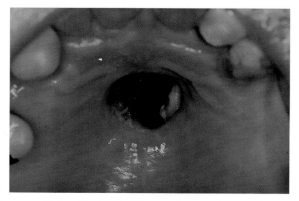

FIG. 1–110. Palatal lesion in Wegener's granulomatosis

■ Epidermolysis Bullosa

This is a generic term that includes several genetically derived bullous subtypes and one acquired subtype. Autoantibodies to type VII collagen are associated with the acquired type. No circulating antibodies are seen in the hereditary forms.

Large flaccid bullae are seen in areas of pressure in all forms of this condition (Figs. 1–107 and 1–108). The severity of the disease is markedly greater in the recessive forms. Nails and teeth may be dystrophic. Because of perioral scarring, constriction of the oral orifice is seen, making access for dental care difficult. Ultrastructure characterizes the disease subtypes. Bulla formation is in a subepithelial location.

■ Midline Granuloma and Wegener's Granulomatosis

These are two etiologically different diseases with similar clinical expression. Both are of unknown etiology and result in destructive lesions of the midline upper respiratory tract.

Midline granuloma typically affects the hard palate and adjacent nasal region. There may be perforation of the nasal septum, hard palate, and blood vessels. Microscopically, the process appears as nonspecific acute and chronic inflammation with necrosis (Fig. 1–109). Many cases represent occult lymphoma. Diagnosis is difficult both clinically and microscopically: typically, several biopsies are taken before a definitive diagnosis is made. The disease must be separated from Wegener's granulomatosis, tertiary syphilis, and malignancy, especially lymphoma. Radiation is generally effective in controlling this mysterious "inflammatory" process.

Wegener's granulomatosis may affect the upper respiratory tract, lung, and kidney. The nose and palate (Fig. 1–110) may be affected, and occasionally the gingiva. The destructive lesions consist of necrotizing vasculitis and granulomatous inflammation (Fig. 1–111). Respiratory and renal failure are consequences of lung and kidney lesions. Chemotherapy (cyclophosphamide and corticosteroids) has been effective in controlling this disease.

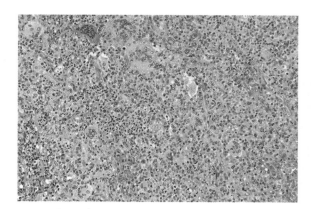

FIG. 1–111. Granulomatous reaction in Wegener's granulomatosis

CHAPTER 2

White-Yellow Lesions

Hereditary-Congenital

Leukoedema

White Sponge Nevus

Fordyce Granules

Reactive

Frictional Hyperkeratosis

Snuff Dipper's Pouch

Nicotine Stomatitis

Actinic Cheilitis

Submucous Fibrosis

Dentifrice Injury

Immune Dysfunction

Lichen Planus

Opportunistic Infections

Hairy Leukoplakia

Candidiasis

Idiopathic

Idiopathic Leukoplakia

Geographic Tongue

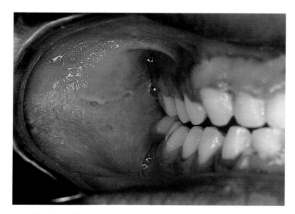

FIG. 2–1. Leukoedema

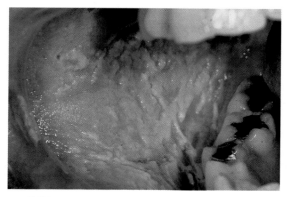

FIG. 2–2. White sponge nevus

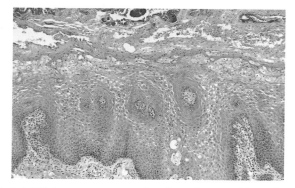

FIG. 2–3. White sponge nevus showing edema and hyperkeratosis

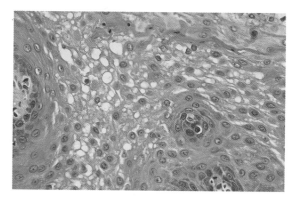

FIG. 2–4. White sponge nevus showing perinuclear condensation

■ Leukoedema

This is a uniform opacification of the buccal mucosa due to intracellular edema (Fig. 2–1). It is a common phenomenon that many believe to be a variation of normal. The condition cannot be removed with simple scraping, but it can be reduced in intensity by stretching the cheek. Other than to differentiate this bilateral white condition from white sponge nevus, hereditary benign intraepithelial dyskeratosis, and cheek chewing, it has no significance.

■ White Sponge Nevus

This is an autosomal dominant condition that has been attributed to mutations in keratin 4 and/or 13 genes. The lesion appears as bilateral white spongy or folded buccal mucosa that extends into the sulcular tissue (Fig. 2–2). Other oral sites, as well as other mucosal regions, may be similarly affected. Microscopically, tissue shows marked epithelial edema with a characteristic perinuclear condensation of eosinophilic keratin (Figs. 2–3 and 2–4).

Differential diagnosis includes other bilateral white lesions, such as cheek chewing, leukoedema, lichen planus, and *hereditary benign intraepithelial dyskeratosis* (HBID). The latter condition is also a hereditary phenomenon (autosomal dominant) that has been described in a small triracial isolate in North Carolina. It results clinically in bilateral white spongy lesions of the buccal mucosa and contiguous structures. It also affects the eye, resulting in irritating periodic hyperplastic epithelial plaques. HBID is microscopically different from white sponge nevus by the formation of numerous separate intraepithelial dyskeratotic keratinocytes. Neither white sponge nevus nor HBID has malignant potential.

■ Fordyce Granules

Fordyce granules represent ectopic sebaceous glands in mucous membranes. This is a common occurrence in the buccal mucosa and lip, although other sites may be affected (Fig. 2–5). Its only significance lies in its differentiation from other white-yellow mucosal lesions. Diagnosis can usually be made on clinical appearance alone.

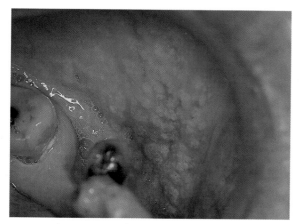

FIG. 2–5. Fordyce granules in buccal mucosa

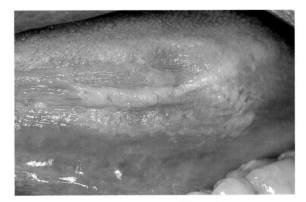

FIG. 2–6. Frictional hyperkeratosis of lateral tongue

■ Frictional Hyperkeratosis

White patches resulting from chronic friction or irritation are common oral mucosal lesions (Figs. 2–6 through 2–9). They are somewhat analogous to a callus occurring on the skin in response to chronic low-grade irritation.

ETIOLOGY

A cause-and-effect relationship should be evident for these lesions. Chronic rubbing or friction stimulates the production of keratin in the area. If there is no obvious cause, white patches should be regarded as idiopathic and managed as such.

CLINICAL FEATURES

Frictional hyperkeratosis occurs in areas that are easily and commonly traumatized, such as the lower lip, lateral margins of the tongue, and buccal mucosa (Fig. 2–6). Also, edentulous alveolar ridges that are used for mastication also show this hyperkeratotic change. *Cheek chewing* is a form of frictional hyperkeratosis and appears as a flat or possibly shaggy white lesion from the angle of the mouth along the occlusal line to the molar region (Figs. 2–7 and 2–8).

MICROSCOPIC FEATURES

Epithelium shows a normal maturation pattern with excessive surface keratin (Fig. 2–9). Keratin may be parakeratin or orthokeratin. There should be no keratinocyte atypia. Inflammatory cell infiltrates are variable.

TREATMENT

Biopsy may not be necessary if the cause of the lesion is obvious. Elimination of the habit or causative agent should result in improvement of the lesion. If there is a question about the cause, biopsy is indicated.

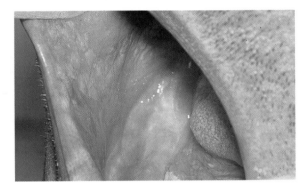

FIG. 2–7. Hyperkeratosis in a cigarette smoker and cheek chewer

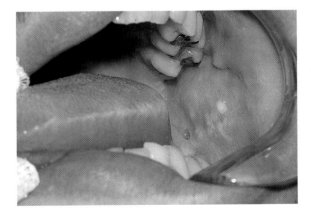

FIG. 2–8. Hyperkeratosis in a tongue and cheek chewer

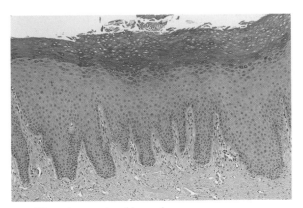

FIG. 2–9. Hyperkeratosis of buccal mucosa

CHAPTER 2: White-Yellow Lesions ■ *Reactive*

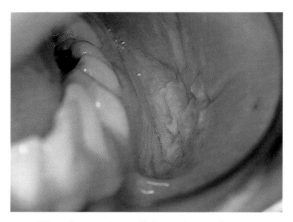

FIG. 2–10. Hyperkeratotic snuff dipper's pouch

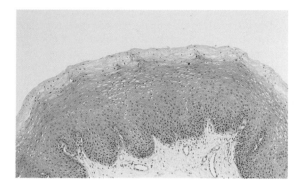

FIG. 2–11. Edema and parakeratosis in snuff pouch

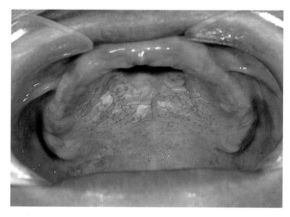

FIG. 2–12. Nicotine stomatitis

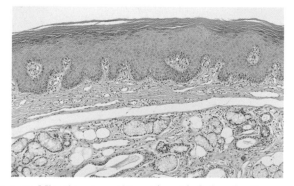

FIG. 2–13. Nicotine stomatitis with epithelial and salivary

■ Snuff Dipper's Pouch

The habitual use of smokeless tobacco in any form eventually results in a keratinized protective mucosal pouch around the site where the tobacco is held. In addition to increasing one's risk for oral cancer, smokeless tobacco can result in acceleration of periodontal disease, dental abrasion, and alterations in taste and smell.

Finely divided tobacco or snuff appears to be more likely to cause opacification of mucous membrane than larger-cut chewing tobacco. The cause-and-effect relationship is obvious. The tissue changes are believed to be in response to the tobacco itself and possibly to flavoring agents or moisture retention factors. The pH of snuff may also contribute to the tissue changes.

Clinically, lesions associated with smokeless tobacco first appear as erythema. Eventually the mucosa becomes hyperkeratotic or white and has a granular or wrinkled appearance (Fig. 2–10). The lesion is painless and is discovered by either the patient or the clinician on routine oral examination. Most lesions are in the mandibular mucobuccal fold adjacent to incisors or molars.

Microscopically, parakeratosis is usually seen, as is intracellular edema (Fig. 2–11). Although dysplasia is possible, it is uncommon. Subjacent salivary glands show inflammatory change.

Elimination of the habit typically eliminates the lesion. Persistent white or red patches should be biopsied. The risk of malignant change, especially to verrucous carcinoma, increases with long-term use.

■ Nicotine Stomatitis

This is another relatively common tobacco-related white lesion associated with pipe, cigar, and cigarette smoking. Unless the habit is particularly intense or the patient is a reverse smoker, the risk for malignant change is apparently quite low.

The combination of tobacco smoke and heat of combustion is believed to be important in this tissue change. The intensity of these factors is markedly increased with reverse smoking and significantly adds to the risk of malignant transformation.

Clinically, tissue changes occur predominantly in the palate and appear as a generalized white opacification (Fig. 2–12). Salivary gland ducts, which become inflamed, appear as red dots in this opacified tissue.

Microscopically, surface epithelium exhibits hyperkeratosis (Fig. 2–13). Underlying salivary glands show inflammatory change with squamous metaplasia of excretory ducts.

Elimination of the habit should cause significant reversal of the palatal tissue changes. Risk of malignancy is reduced; however, conditioning of the rest of the oral cavity and upper respiratory tract by the tobacco smoke is of continued concern.

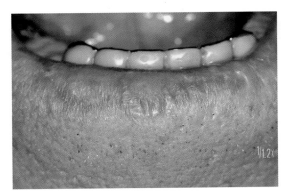

FIG. 2–14. Actinic cheilitis

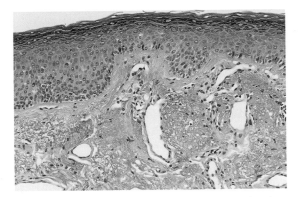

FIG. 2–15. Actinic cheilitis, highlighted by basophilic change

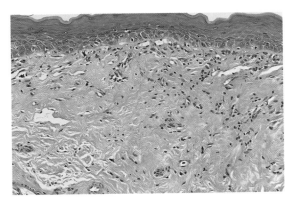

FIG. 2–16. Submucous fibrosis

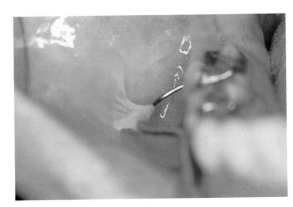

FIG. 2–17. Dentifrice-associated slough

■ Actinic Cheilitis

Solar cheilitis results from the effects of ultraviolet light on exposed vermilion and skin. This is due predominantly to UVB light. The effects are seen predominantly on the lower lip and consist of epithelial atrophy, opacification due to keratosis, wrinkling from elastosis, and reduced definition of the skin line (Figs. 2–14 and 2–15). Microscopically, epithelial atrophy, hyperkeratosis, basophilic change of collagen, and telangiectasias are seen. The effects of ultraviolet light are permanent but can be retarded with use of sunscreens and sun blocks. Solar cheilitis is at risk for malignant transformation to squamous cell carcinoma. Nonhealing ulceration and induration should mandate biopsy.

■ Submucous Fibrosis

Submucous fibrosis is a chronic process in which progressive scarring provides a light color to the mucosa. It is rarely seen in the United States but is common in Southeast Asia and India, where tobacco habits include the use of betel nut. This condition is believed to be closely related to the use of this material and possibly to other dietary factors. The submucosal scarring occurs predominantly in the buccal mucosa, soft palate, and contiguous sites. The tissue loses elasticity and may result in trismus and a constricted oral orifice.

Microscopically, there is epithelial atrophy and occasionally dysplasia (Fig. 2–16). Submucosa becomes hyalinized as the collagen content increases. The permanent scarring associated with this phenomenon is difficult to treat. Corticosteroids and surgical procedures have been used with some success. There is significant risk of malignant transformation to squamous cell carcinoma.

■ Dentifrice Injury

Substances used in dentifrices have on occasion been linked to superficial slough of mucosal keratin (Fig. 2–17). This trivial change can be eliminated by the use of a bland toothpaste. There are no known ill effects associated with this phenomenon. Recently, some investigators have observed white mucosal changes, especially in the maxillary vestibule, that are believed to be related to the use of toothpaste and mouthwash containing the substance sanguinaria (Fig. 2–18).

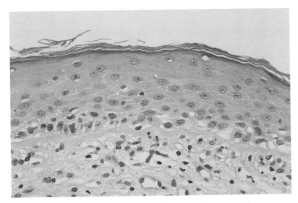

FIG. 2–18. Sanguinaria-associated keratosis, maxillary vestibule

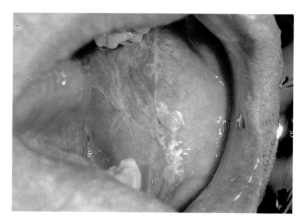

FIG. 2–19. Lichen planus, reticular form

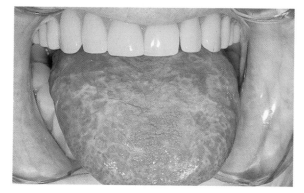

FIG. 2–20. Lichen planus, reticular form

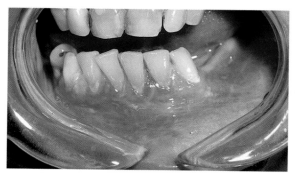

FIG. 2–21. Lichen planus, atrophic form

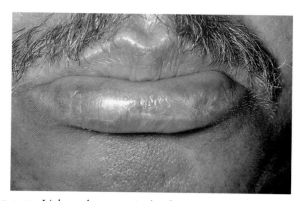

FIG. 2–22. Lichen planus, reticular form

■ Lichen Planus

Lichen planus is a relatively common chronic disease that may affect the skin and/or mucous membrane. It typically presents bilaterally in the buccal mucosa and is steroid-responsive. The cause is unknown.

ETIOLOGY AND PATHOGENESIS

Lichen planus is believed to be related to an abnormal cell-mediated immune response. The trigger of this process is unknown. Recruitment and retention of T lymphocytes to mucosal and skin sites appears to be a requisite event in the development of this disease. Vascular adhesion molecules are known to be overexpressed in lichen planus tissue and are believed to result in recruitment of lymphocytes (Fig. 2–28). These and other immune cells, such as macrophages, factor XIIIa dendrocytes, and Langerhans cells, are thought to be the primary sources of the proinflammatory cytokines that seem to be fueling this process. The recruited T cells appear to mediate basal cell death through the triggering of apoptosis. When basal cell death is extensive, epithelium may be lost, resulting in ulcerative or erosive lichen planus.

CLINICAL FEATURES

Lichen planus typically affects middle-aged men and women. Most patients are unaware of oral lichen planus unless it is the erosive or atrophic type, in which case the patient experiences pain in the affected site. Cutaneous lichen planus, which affects the lower legs, forearms, and scalp, appears as red to violaceous papules that are pruritic.

The most common oral type of lichen planus is the reticular form in which there are interlacing white lines (Wickham's striae) (Fig. 2–19). Buccal mucosa is most frequently involved, characteristically bilaterally and symmetrically. Other sites may be affected, especially the tongue, gingiva, and lips (Figs. 2–20 through 2–22). Any of these areas may be ulcerated, resulting in erosive lichen planus (Fig. 2–23). There is an atrophic form of lichen planus (usually gingiva) in which the lesions appear predominantly red with only delicate white striae (see Fig. 2–21). A plaque form is infrequently seen (Fig. 2–24), and a bullous form is rarely encountered.

MICROSCOPIC FEATURES

Three criteria are critical to the diagnosis of lichen planus: (1) hyperkeratosis, (2) basal layer vacuolization with keratinocyte apoptosis, and (3) a lymphophagocytic infiltrate at the epithelial–connective tissue interface (Figs. 2–25 through 2–27). Direct immunofluorescence shows deposition of fibrinogen along the basement membrane zone.

TREATMENT

Treatment strategies are directed toward control rather than cure. Corticosteroids, either topical or systemic, provide significant change in the appearance of the disease; however, the condition is likely to rebound after the discontinuation of the corticosteroid. In severe cases of erosive lichen planus, the use of prednisone, with or without steroid-sparing drugs, is justified. Although controversial, most investigators believe that oral lichen planus increases the patient's risk, although by only a small amount, for squamous cell carcinoma. Differential diagnostic considerations include lichenoid drug reaction, lupus erythematosus, cheek chewing, and candidiasis.

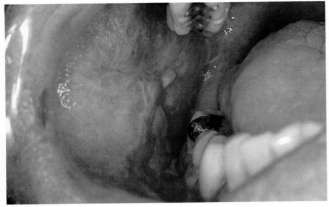

FIG. 2–23. Lichen planus, erosive (ulcerative) type

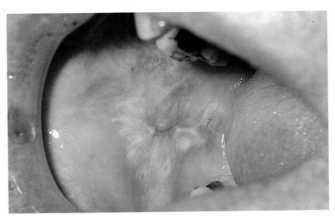

FIG. 2–24. Lichen planus, plaque type

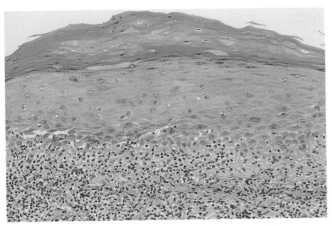

FIG. 2–25. Lichen planus showing keratosis and infiltrate

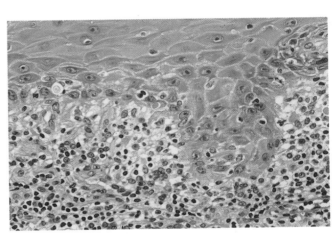

FIG. 2–26. High magnification of Figure 2–25

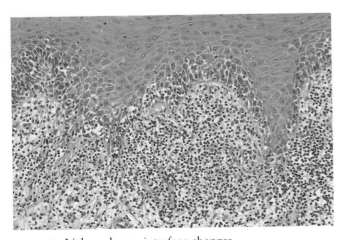

FIG. 2–27. Lichen planus, interface changes

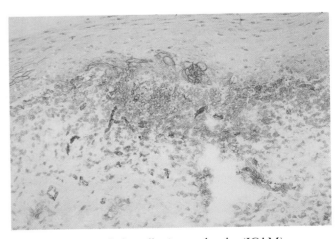

FIG. 2–28. Stain (red) for adhesion molecules (ICAM)

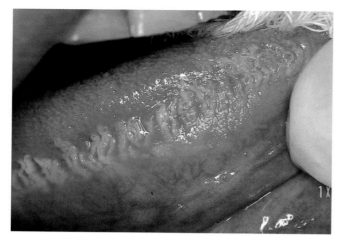

FIG. 2–29. Hairy leukoplakia

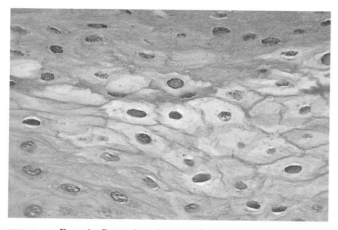

FIG. 2–30. Epstein-Barr virus intranuclear changes in hairy leukoplakia

■ Hairy Leukoplakia

This white plaque, usually seen on the lateral surfaces of the tongue, was originally described in AIDS and pre-AIDS patients. Subsequently, however, it has occurred in other immunosuppressed patients and rarely in immuno-competent patients.

ETIOLOGY AND PATHOGENESIS

Hairy leukoplakia is an opportunistic infection caused by Epstein-Barr virus. In the HIV population, where it is most frequently seen, its prevalence is approximately 20% in HIV-infected individuals and rises to as high as 80% in AIDS patients. There is an inverse relationship with the peripheral CD4 count. Medically immunosuppressed patients (transplant patients) may also develop this lesion.

CLINICAL FEATURES

This white lesion may be bilateral or unilateral on the lateral margins of the tongue (Fig. 2–29). Rarely, it is seen in the buccal mucosa or the floor of the mouth. The lesion may be colonized by *Candida albicans*. The surface architecture ranges from flat to "hairy," in which there are numerous small keratotic projections.

MICROSCOPIC FEATURES

The key diagnostic feature of hairy leukoplakia is evidence of intranuclear viral inclusions in upper-level keratinocytes (Fig. 2–30). This may be in the form of nuclear smudging with peripherally displaced chromatin in a beaded or necklace type pattern, or distinct eosinophilic inclusions. Other architectural features of hairy leukoplakia include parakeratosis, "balloon cell" or edematous changes of upper-level keratinocytes, and a general paucity of inflammatory cells and Langerhans cells (Fig. 2–31). *In situ* hybridization for Epstein-Barr virus can be used to confirm histologic findings if necessary (Fig. 2–32).

TREATMENT

No specific treatment is required. However, if it is objectionable to the patient, the lesion does respond to acyclovir and vitamin A derivatives. Differential diagnosis includes idiopathic leukoplakia and tongue chewing. Biopsy is diagnostic.

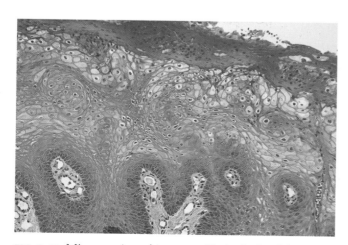

FIG. 2–31. Microscopic architecture of hairy leukoplakia

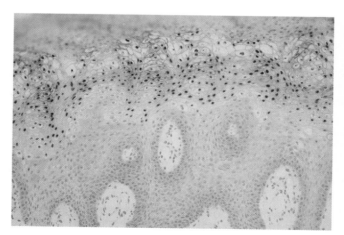

FIG. 2–32. Positive nuclear signal (blue) for Epstein-Barr virus in hairy leukoplakia

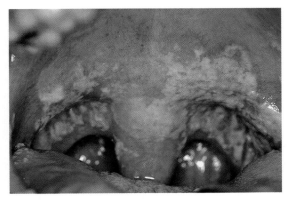

FIG. 2–33. Acute candidiasis in HIV-positive patient

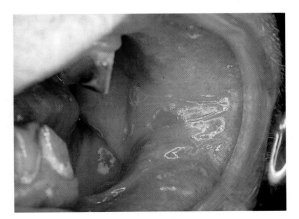

FIG. 2–34. Acute candidiasis in a radiation patient

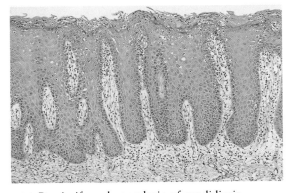

FIG. 2–35. Psoriasiform hyperplasia of candidiasis

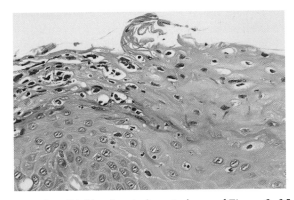

FIG. 2–36. Candidal hyphae in keratin layer of Figure 2–35

■ Candidiasis

Oral candidiasis is an opportunistic infection by *Candida albicans*, although other species may produce this condition. There are several clinical forms of candidiasis that are categorized by the region affected and the clinical presentation.

ETIOLOGY AND PATHOGENESIS

Candida albicans is a resident of the normal oral flora in a large segment of the population. It can become pathogenic when one of several predisposing factors is present. These factors most commonly include antibiotic therapy, corticosteroid therapy, xerostomia, diabetes mellitus, chemotherapy or radiation therapy, poor oral hygiene, and immunosuppression.

CLINICAL FEATURES

Oral candidiasis can be classified into acute, chronic, and mucocutaneous forms. The acute form, sometimes called *thrush* (fungal colonies), presents as soft white nodules on mucous membranes (Figs. 2–33 and 2–34). Removal of these plaques or nodules results in a raw, bleeding surface. Any site may be affected, but the palate and buccal mucosa seem to be favored.

Chronic candidiasis presents as red patches with no obvious surface colonies. This may be seen in the palate under a poorly fitting denture (*denture sore mouth*). It may present as cracking and fissuring of the angle of the mouth, known as *angular cheilitis* or *perlèche*. A lesion in the midline of the tongue anterior to the circumvallate papillae, known as *median rhomboid glossitis*, is another form of chronic candidiasis. Also, it may present as a generalized red atrophic tongue, especially in women. Chronic hypertrophic candidiasis is a subtype that appears as a keratotic plaque containing fungus, usually near the angle of the mouth in the buccal mucosa.

Mucocutaneous candidiasis, as the name implies, affects the mucous membranes, skin, and nails. Subsets of mucocutaneous candidiasis include a familial form and a syndrome that includes myositis and thymoma.

MICROSCOPIC FEATURES

In the acute form, fungal hyphae can be shown in scrapings of the lesions. They can also be demonstrated in keratin layers of biopsy specimens. Fungal hyphae are more difficult to demonstrate in chronic candidiasis. However, in this form a psoriasiform hyperplasia is seen microscopically, usually with a neutrophilic infiltrate of superficial keratin (Figs. 2–35 and 2–36).

TREATMENT

Topical application of various forms of nystatin or clotrimazole is effective in treating acute candidiasis. Chronic candidiasis may also be treated in a similar manner but requires an extended period of therapy. Of paramount importance are the recognition and control of predisposing factors. In more difficult cases, such as patients who are immunosuppressed, systemic administration of other drugs such as amphotericin B, ketoconazole, fluconazole, or itraconazole may be required.

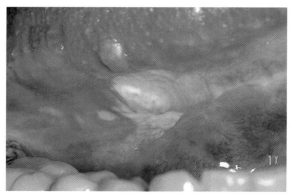

FIG. 2–37. Idiopathic leukoplakia of lateral-ventral tongue

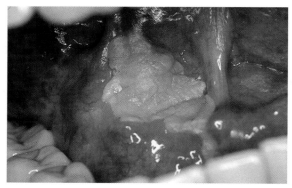

FIG. 2–38. Idiopathic leukoplakia of floor of mouth

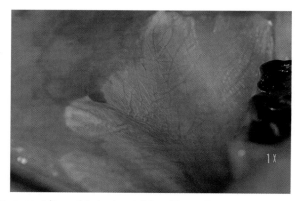

FIG. 2–39. Idiopathic leukoplakia of buccal mucosa

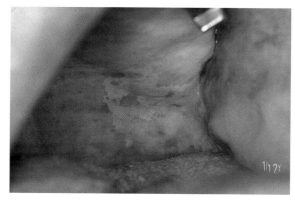

FIG. 2–40. Idiopathic leukoplakia of palate

■ Idiopathic Leukoplakia

Idiopathic leukoplakia is a clinical term used to describe a white patch that cannot be rubbed off and cannot be designated as any other clinically diagnostic condition. The cause of these mysterious patches is unknown, and their significance lies in the fact that a small percentage show premalignant or malignant epithelial change and a small percentage eventually become malignant (squamous cell carcinoma).

ETIOLOGY AND PATHOGENESIS
Tobacco in any form is believed to be associated with the development of some of these lesions. Other factors that have been cited as possibly playing a pathogenetic role include alcohol, trauma, *Candida albicans*, and nutritional deficiencies.

CLINICAL FEATURES
This lesion typically occurs in middle-aged and older adults. It is painless. Although it may be seen in any region of the mouth, the lateral tongue and the floor of the mouth are considered high-risk sites (Figs. 2–37 through 2–41). The opacity of these lesions varies from slight to marked, in which there is considerable keratin production by the lesion. Although the range of malignancy and malignant transformation in these lesions is quite variable depending on the world population studied, approximately 5% are malignant at first biopsy and another 5% develop into malignancy at a later date (Fig. 2–42).

A subset of idiopathic leukoplakia, known as *proliferative verrucous leukoplakia*, develops in multiple sites, is persistent, and eventually becomes verruciform in profile (see Chap. 4). Malignant transformation to verrucous or squamous cell carcinoma is seen in as many as 15% of cases.

MICROSCOPIC FEATURES
The histologic spectrum for idiopathic leukoplakia ranges from hyperkeratosis to invasive squamous cell carcinoma (Figs. 2–43 through 2–45). Changes at the lesion edge can often be abrupt (Figs. 2–46 and 2–47). Because the microscopic diagnosis cannot be predicted from the clinical appearance, all cases of idiopathic leukoplakia must be biopsied. Most lesions will, in fact, be simple hyperkeratosis, but at risk for progressive change. Overexpression of p53 protein has been described in dysplastic lesions (Fig. 2–48). Mutations of *p53* gene appear to occur late in the transformation of dysplasia to carcinoma.

TREATMENT
Generally, once the diagnosis is established, lesions showing moderate or more severe change should be completely excised. Recurrence after any type of surgical removal is not uncommon.

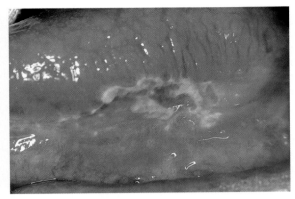

FIG. 2–41. Idiopathic leukoplakia of lateral tongue

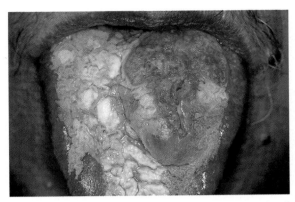

FIG. 2–42. Carcinoma developing in idiopathic leukoplakia

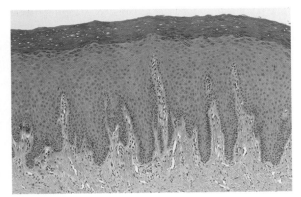

FIG. 2–43. Hyperkeratosis (idiopathic leukoplakia)

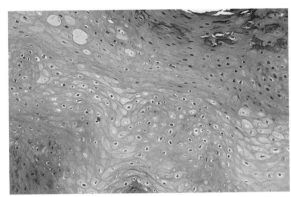

FIG. 2–44. Edema and parakeratosis (idiopathic leukoplakia)

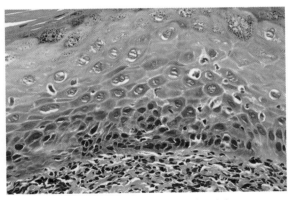

FIG. 2–45. Dysplasia in idiopathic leukoplakia

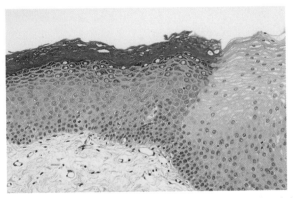

FIG. 2–46. Abrupt change to hyperkeratosis in leukoplakia

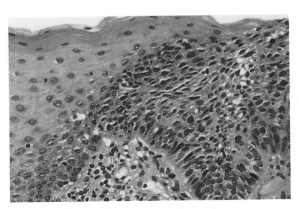

FIG. 2–47. Abrupt change to *in situ* carcinoma

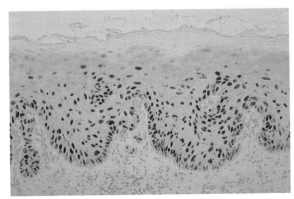

FIG. 2–48. Positive p53 stain in dysplasia (idiopathic leuko-plakia)

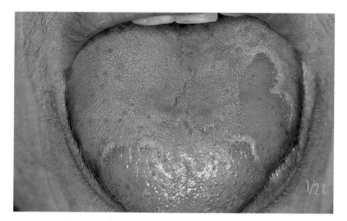
FIG. 2-49. Geographic tongue

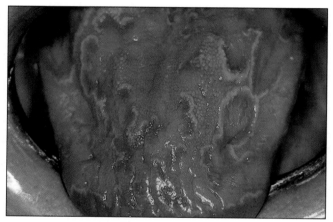
FIG. 2-50. Geographic tongue

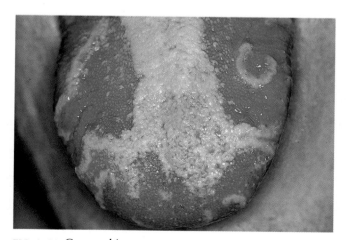
FIG. 2-51. Geographic tongue

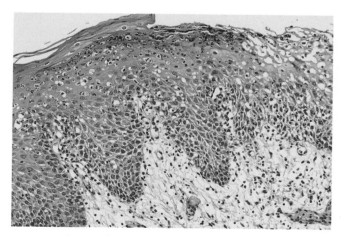
FIG. 2-52. Geographic tongue, keratosis left and atrophy right

■ Geographic Tongue

Also known as *benign migratory glossitis*, this condition of unknown cause is a dynamic process that changes pattern with time. This is a relatively common self-limiting condition that is usually asymptomatic and is of no consequence.

ETIOLOGY
Attempts to link this disease to stress and infection have been futile. It has been suggested, but not confirmed, as being a manifestation of psoriasis. The association may be coincidental because of the relative prevalences of geographic tongue and psoriasis.

CLINICAL FEATURES
The tongue is almost always the affected site (Figs. 2–49 through 2–51), although it has been described in the buccal mucosa and lip. Patches of atrophic epithelium are surrounded by hyperkeratotic margins. Ulceration is not seen. Patients are usually asymptomatic, although some may complain of pain and sensitivity to some foods. Followed over time, the atrophic and keratotic areas migrate across the surface of the tongue, producing a slightly different pattern. Lesions may completely disappear and return at a later date. Some patients indicate that their exacerbations are related to emotional stress.

MICROSCOPIC FEATURES
The areas of redness are associated with loss of papillae and the appearance of neutrophils and lymphocytes within and subjacent to the epithelium (Fig. 2–52). The white marginated areas are predominantly hyperkeratotic, with some lymphocyte infiltration of supporting tissue. Dysplasia is not seen in these lesions, and there is no malignant potential.

TREATMENT
Because the lesions are typically asymptomatic and the disease is self-limited, treatment is not required. Topical corticosteroids may be used to help control lesions that are sensitive or cosmetically objectionable.

Red-Blue-Black Lesions

Vascular Lesions

Kaposi's Sarcoma

Hemangioma

Mucosal Varices

Erythroplakia

Vitamin B Deficiencies and Anemias

Chronic Candidiasis

Pyogenic Granuloma

Peripheral Giant Cell Granuloma

Plasma Cell Gingivitis

Hypersensitivity Reactions

Hereditary Hemorrhagic Telangiectasias

Petechiae and Ecchymoses

Melanocytic Lesions

Physiologic Pigmentation

Oral Melanotic Macule

Smoking-Associated Melanosis

Peutz-Jeghers Syndrome

Addison's Disease

Neuroectodermal Tumor of Infancy

Melanocytic Nevi

Oral Melanoma

Other Pigmented Lesions

Hairy Tongue

Amalgam Tattoo

Pigmentation Associated with Drugs

Postinflammatory Pigmentation

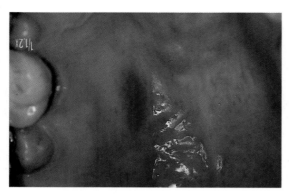

FIG. 3–1. Kaposi's sarcoma, macular stage

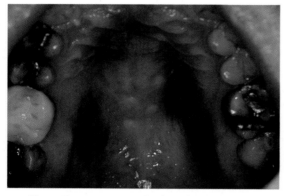

FIG. 3–2. Kaposi's sarcoma, multiple palatal lesions

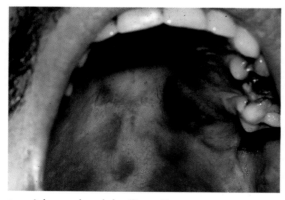

FIG. 3–3. Advanced nodular Kaposi's sarcoma

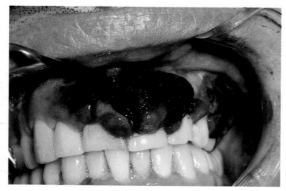

FIG. 3–4. Advanced Kaposi's sarcoma

■ Kaposi's Sarcoma

Kaposi's sarcoma represents a proliferation of predominantly endothelial cells that behaves in some ways like a reactive lesion and in some ways like a malignant neoplasm. It is most commonly associated with immunodeficiency, although rarely it has been described in other clinical settings.

ETIOLOGY AND PATHOGENESIS

Human herpesvirus type 8, also known as Kaposi's sarcoma-associated herpesvirus, has been identified in all forms of Kaposi's sarcoma and is believed to be in large part responsible for the development of these lesions. Its effects are believed to be associated with focal release of cytokines and growth factors that fuel the proliferative process. These proinflammatory and proliferative substances are derived from the endothelial cells themselves, as well as recruited macrophages, lymphocytes, and dendrocytes. The products of HIV infection, such as TAT protein, are also believed to be responsible for the mediation of this process.

CLINICAL FEATURES

The classic Mediterranean type and the endemic type of Kaposi's sarcoma rarely affect the oral mucosa. The immunodeficiency type, which is seen in organ transplant patients and particularly AIDS patients, commonly has oral expression. Lesions are initially macular and with time become nodular and bulky (Figs. 3–1 through 3–4). Oral lesions are frequently multifocal and are most commonly seen in the palate, gingiva, and tongue. Oral lesions may precede cutaneous lesions, or they may be the only expression of this disease. The incidence of Kaposi's sarcoma in AIDS patients has declined in recent years, presumably due to the effects of chemotherapeutic agents used to treat AIDS.

MICROSCOPIC FEATURES

The early or macular lesions of oral Kaposi's sarcoma appear as hypercellular foci in connective tissue (Figs. 3–5 and 3–6). Bland-appearing spindle cells form ill-defined vascular channels with red cell extravasation. Advanced lesions show a marked increase in spindle cells and abundant atypical vascular channels (Fig. 3–7). Hyaline globules, representing red blood cell breakdown, may also be seen (Fig. 3–8). Immunohistochemical stains of Kaposi's sarcoma show CD34-positive endothelial cells (Fig. 3–9) in company with large numbers of macrophages (Fig. 3–10), lymphocytes, and dendrocytes. A clinically and microscopically similar bacterial infection caused by *Bartonella henselae* or *B. quintana*, known as bacillary angiomatosis, has been described in skin, but only rarely in oral mucosa.

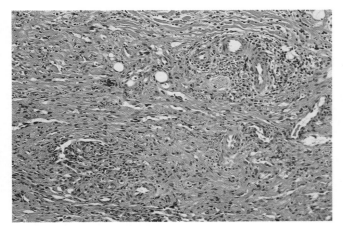

FIG. 3–5. Early or macular Kaposi's sarcoma

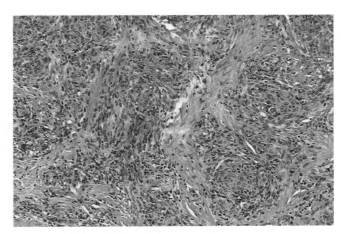

FIG. 3–6. Advanced Kaposi's sarcoma

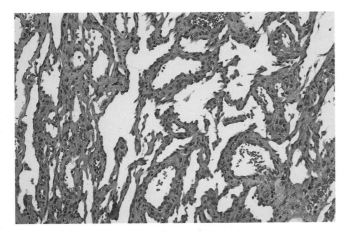

FIG. 3–7. Bizarre vessels in advanced Kaposi's sarcoma

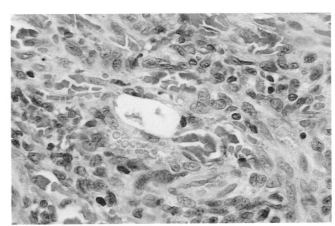

FIG. 3–8. Hyaline globules in Kaposi's sarcoma

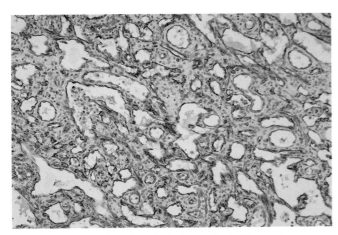

FIG. 3–9. Positive CD34 endothelial cells in Kaposi's sarcoma

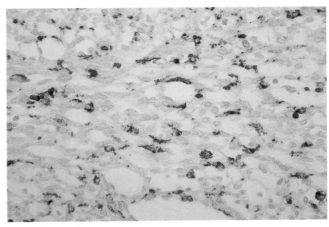

FIG. 3–10. Positive-stained (CD68) macrophages in Kaposi's sarcoma

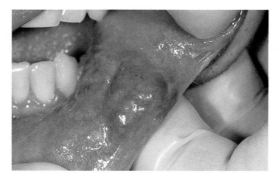

FIG. 3–11. Vascular malformation of lip and buccal mucosa

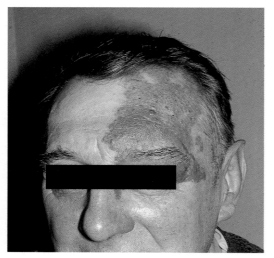

FIG. 3–12. Vascular malformation in Sturge-Weber syndrome

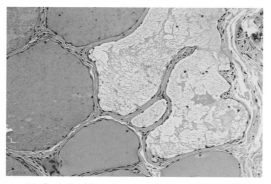

FIG. 3–13. Endothelial-lined spaces in vascular malformation

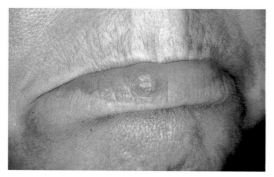

FIG. 3–14. Varix of lower lip

■ Hemangioma

Hemangioma is a generic term that includes congenital hemangiomas and other vascular malformations.

The congenital hemangioma, or *strawberry nevus*, appears on skin at or shortly after birth. After a seemingly rapid growth phase, most lesions involute. Those that persist may be circumscribed so that surgical removal is feasible.

The more problematic lesions, vascular malformations, are present at or after the time of birth and enlarge as the patient grows. These lesions are persistent and poorly circumscribed. They may affect skin, mucous membrane, and bone (Fig. 3–11). Eradication is generally difficult, and recurrences are common after excision. These lesions, unlike congenital hemangioma, may produce a bruit or thrill.

A subset of vascular malformation is *Sturge-Weber syndrome (encephalotrigeminal angiomatosis)* (Fig. 3–12). This syndrome includes vascular malformations of the meninges and face, usually in an area innervated by one of the branches of the trigeminal nerve. Mental retardation and seizures are also part of the syndrome. The vascular lesion of this syndrome is sometimes called *port-wine stain* or *nevus flammeus*. Port-wine stains can also be seen as isolated lesions not associated with this syndrome.

On microscopy, congenital hemangiomas consist of either small capillaries or larger cavernous spaces lined by endothelium. There appears to be no significance relative to the size of these vascular channels. Vascular malformations represent combinations of capillaries and other larger vascular channels (Fig. 3–13).

■ Mucosal Varices

Varicose veins are commonly seen in the ventral tongue, representing congenital enlargement of these vascular channels. Acquired varices develop frequently in the lower lips of sun-damaged tissues (Fig. 3–14). These vascular malformations blanch on compression and on occasion undergo thrombosis (Fig. 3–15). The thrombotic event is of no significance in this site.

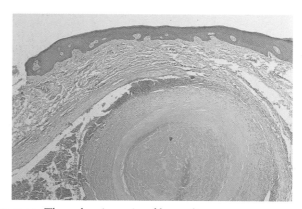

FIG. 3–15. Thrombus in varix of lower lip

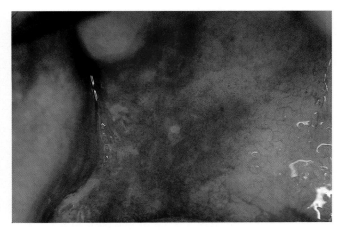

FIG. 3–16. Erythroplakia of soft palate

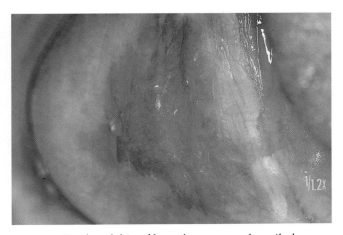

FIG. 3–17. Erythroplakia of buccal mucosa and vestibule

■ Erythroplakia

Oral erythroplakia is a clinical term that refers to an idiopathic red patch. Most of these lesions represent dysplasia or carcinoma.

ETIOLOGY

The cause of this lesion is unknown, but factors responsible for oral cancer are also believed to be responsible for erythroplakias. Therefore, tobacco probably plays the most significant role in the induction of these lesions.

CLINICAL FEATURES

Erythroplakia is much less frequently seen than its white, or leukoplakia, counterpart. It presents as a relatively distinct red patch, and causative factors are usually not evident. It may be seen in any site (Figs. 3–16 and 3–17). High-risk sites are the floor of the mouth, tongue, and retromolar pad. This is a condition of older individuals, usually over age 50. There is a penile equivalent known as erythroplasia of Queyrat.

MICROSCOPIC FEATURES

Approximately 90% of these lesions are at least severe dysplasia. Many represent *in situ* carcinomas (Fig. 3–18) and squamous cell carcinomas. The floor of the mouth in particular may show surface changes that extend into the excretory ducts of the subjacent salivary glands (Fig. 3–19).

TREATMENT

Treatment is based on the definitive microscopic diagnosis. The strategy should be to eliminate dysplastic red lesions if surgically feasible. *In situ* carcinomas should be excised with wide margins. If biopsy shows extension into excretory ducts, the lesion should be treated as a superficially invasive squamous cell carcinoma.

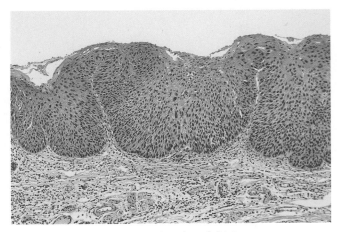

FIG. 3–18. Carcinoma *in situ* (erythroplakia)

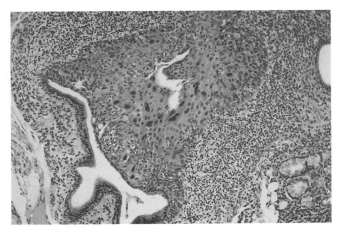

FIG. 3–19. *In situ* carcinoma extending into salivary duct

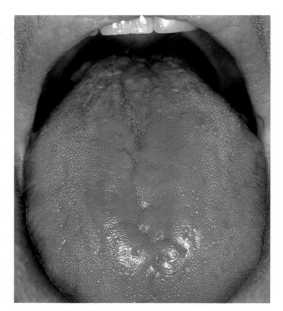

FIG. 3–20. Atrophic glossitis

■ Vitamin B Deficiencies and Anemias

Deficiency of one or more of the B-complex vitamins may result in changes of the oral mucosa. These deficiencies are likely to be related to malnutrition associated with alcoholism, starvation, or fad diets. Malabsorption syndromes may also contribute to a deficiency.

Oral signs of this problem include cracking and fissuring at the angles of the mouth (angular cheilitis) and atrophic glossitis. The tongue changes appear as a generalized redness due to atrophy of the papillae (Fig. 3–20). With this change comes pain and burning. Anemias, in particular pernicious anemia and iron deficiency anemia, may result in similar oral changes. Diagnosis of vitamin B deficiencies and anemias is made on the basis of historical, clinical, and laboratory findings. Replacement therapy results in a return of the tissues to a normal state.

■ Chronic Candidiasis

Caused by the fungus *Candida albicans*, chronic candidiasis appears as a red lesion in which fungus is difficult to demonstrate, both clinically and microscopically. Identification of predisposing factors is important in the diagnosis of this condition. Examples of chronic candidiasis include *denture sore mouth*, associated with ill-fitting dentures (Fig. 3–21); *median rhomboid glossitis*, previously regarded as persistence of the embryonic tuberculum impar (Fig. 3–22); and *angular cheilitis* or *perlèche* (Fig. 3–23). Angular cheilitis is frequently coinfected with *Staphylococcus aureus*. Chronic candidiasis tends to be more resistant to therapy than acute candidiasis, although satisfactory results can be achieved with long-term (4 weeks or more) antifungal therapy and correction of underlying predisposing factors.

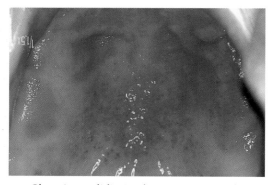

FIG. 3–21. Chronic candidiasis (denture sore mouth)

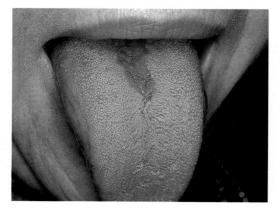

FIG. 3–22. Median rhomboid glossitis (chronic candidiasis)

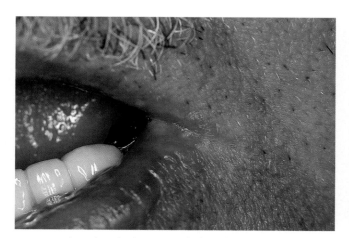

FIG. 3–23. Angular cheilitis or perlèche (chronic candidiasis)

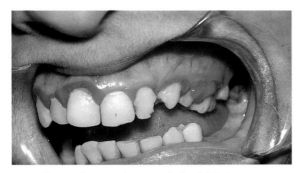

FIG. 3–24. Pyogenic granuloma and gingivitis in pregnant patient

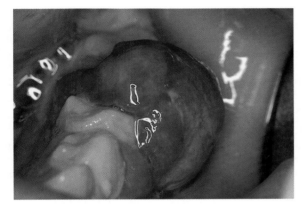

FIG. 3–25. Ulcerated pyogenic granuloma

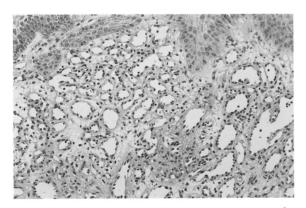

FIG. 3–26. Granulation tissue making up pyogenic granuloma

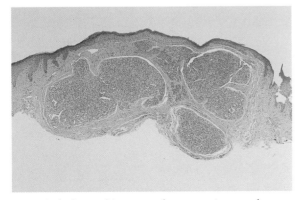

FIG. 3–27. Lobular architecture of a pyogenic granuloma

■ Pyogenic Granuloma

Pyogenic granuloma is a common reactive hyperplasia that is related to trauma or chronic irritation. Lesions are red and appear predominantly in the gingiva, although any commonly traumatized site, such as the lower lip, tongue, and buccal mucosa, may be affected.

ETIOLOGY

This is one of several forms of reactive hyperplasia that occur in oral mucous membranes. It represents overexuberant connective tissue repair to usually a known or suspected stimulus. Calculus, foreign body, and trauma are the usual causative agents. The hormonal changes associated with puberty and pregnancy may contribute to the growth of these lesions. The term "pyogenic granuloma" is a misnomer, as the lesion is neither pus-producing nor granulomatous.

CLINICAL FEATURES

Lesions appear as red masses that are smooth-surfaced or lobulated (Figs. 3–24 and 3–25). Occasionally, the surface becomes ulcerated, resulting in a yellow fibrin-covered ulcer. Females tend to be more frequently affected than males.

MICROSCOPIC FEATURES

Hyperplastic granulation tissue characterizes this lesion (Fig. 3–26). Often lobular masses of granulation tissue can be seen extending into subjacent connective tissue (Figs. 3–27 and 3–28). Inflammatory cells may be seen throughout, especially if there is ulceration. Mitotic figures are often seen.

TREATMENT

Surgical excision is the treatment of choice. Occasionally recurrence is seen, believed to be due to conservative removal. The excision should extend to the periodontal ligament and periosteum. There is no malignant potential for this process.

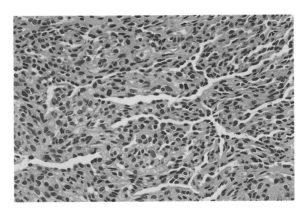

FIG. 3–28. High magnification of Figure 3–27 showing compact vessels

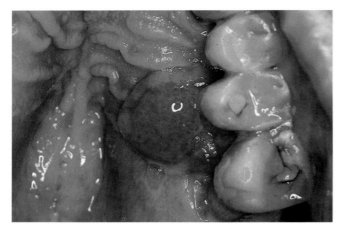

FIG. 3–29. Peripheral giant cell granuloma

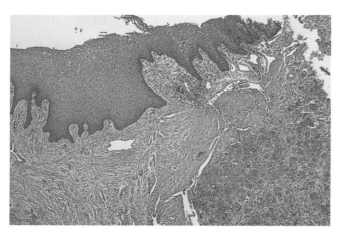

FIG. 3–30. Peripheral giant cell granuloma (right) in mucosa

■ Peripheral Giant Cell Granuloma

This lesion presents as a red to purple mass of the gingiva only. It is one of several common reactive hyperplasias of mucous membrane.

ETIOLOGY
This reactive hyperplasia, like pyogenic granuloma, is believed to represent an overexuberant reaction to chronic irritation. The irritant likely represents a foreign body, calculus, or trauma to the gingiva.

CLINICAL FEATURES
This exclusively gingival lesion typically presents in the tissues that held the succedaneous teeth (alveolus anterior to the first permanent molars) (Fig. 3–29). Females are more often affected than males. It presents as a red to purple mass. When occurring in an edentulous ridge, a subjacent cup-shaped radiolucency may be seen. Slight bone resorption might be seen also with lesions occurring in interdental papillae. Peripheral giant cell granulomas seem to have limited growth potential (approximately 1 cm in diameter).

MICROSCOPIC FEATURES
Fibroblasts make up the substance of these lesions. Abundant numbers of multinucleated giant cells provide a distinctive microscopic picture (Figs. 3–30 and 3–31). The giant cells that characterize this lesion have no known purpose. Their origin may be from fused monocytes recruited from the blood by factors liberated by lesional fibroblasts. Extravasated red cells can be seen throughout, although vessels are not particularly prominent or numerous. Occasionally, islands of new bone can be seen in the center of these lesions.

TREATMENT
Surgical excision is the treatment of choice. Occasional recurrence is seen. Removal to the periosteum or periodontal ligament is recommended. There is no malignant potential. Clinical differential diagnosis would include pyogenic granuloma, parulis (Fig. 3–32), and metastatic neoplasm.

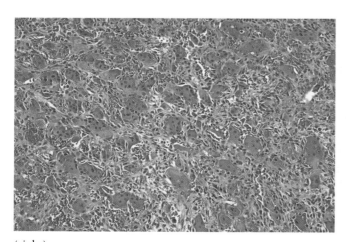

(right)
FIG. 3–31. Peripheral giant cell granuloma

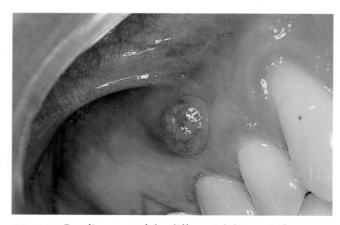

FIG. 3–32. Parulis—part of the differential diagnosis for peripheral giant cell granuloma

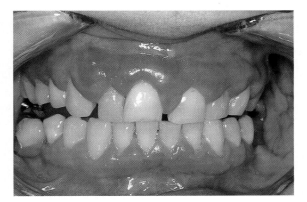

FIG. 3–33. Plasma cell gingivitis

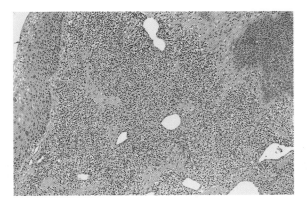

FIG. 3–34. Plasma cell gingivitis

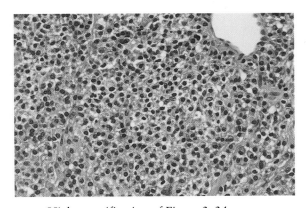

FIG. 3–35. High magnification of Figure 3–34

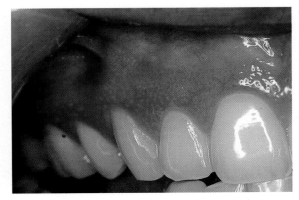

FIG. 3–36. Contact gingivitis

■ Plasma Cell Gingivitis

Patients with plasma cell gingivitis present with enlarged red gingiva. The enlargement is due to an intense reactive plasma cell infiltrate and prominent capillaries.

ETIOLOGY
The intense plasma cell infiltrate seen in this phenomenon is believed to be due to a hyperimmune reaction to an exogenous antigen. Some cases have been linked to a component of chewing gum, mint, or cinnamon. It is not uncommon for the agent to go unidentified.

CLINICAL FEATURES
This infrequently seen condition appears as a boggy red swelling, usually of the entire attached gingiva (Fig. 3–33). Some cases may also show angular cheilitis, and atrophy and fissuring of the tongue. The gingiva may be asymptomatic, but if the tongue and lips are affected, the patient complains of pain.

MICROSCOPIC FEATURES
The most characteristic microscopic finding is an intense infiltrate of mature plasma cells (Figs. 3–34 and 3–35). Surface epithelium may be spongiotic, and Langerhans cells may be prominent. Apoptotic keratinocytes may be seen in the basal and parabasal zone.

DIFFERENTIAL DIAGNOSIS
Differential diagnosis of bright-red gingiva should include, in addition to plasma cell gingivitis, discoid erythematosus, lichen planus, psoriasis, and mucous membrane pemphigoid. Drug and dietary history may be helpful in identifying allergens of etiologic significance.

■ Hypersensitivity Reactions

In addition to plasma cell gingivitis, other hypersensitivity reactions may stimulate a mixed or predominantly lymphocytic response (Figs. 3–36 and 3–37). The associated changes may appear as flat red changes of the gingiva. Other sites, such as lips and tongue, may exhibit similar reddish change. Patients usually complain of sensitivity. Identification of the etiologic agent will require a thorough dietary and drug history. The usual suspects, mint and cinnamon, should be given first consideration.

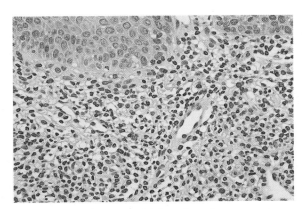

FIG. 3–37. Contact hypersensitivity—lymphocytes and eosinophils

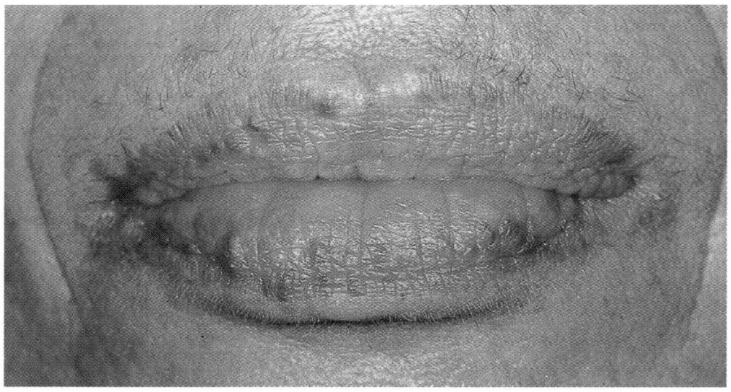

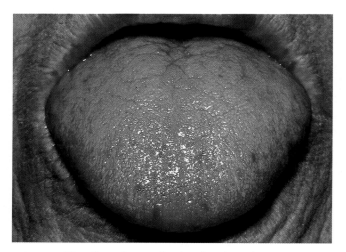

■ Hereditary Hemorrhagic Telangiectasia

Also known as *Rendu-Osler-Weber syndrome*, this rare condition features numerous telangiectasias of the skin, mucous membranes, and occasionally viscera (Figs. 3–38 and 3–39). The condition, which is autosomal dominant, appears early in life and persists through adulthood. The telangiectasias appear as multiple flat or elevated lesions. Lesions in the nasal mucosa may become problematic because of epistaxis. Occasionally, oral or lip lesions may bleed from minor trauma.

FIG. 3–38. Hereditary hemorrhagic telangiectasia

FIG. 3–39. Hereditary hemorrhagic telangiectasia

■ Petechiae and Ecchymoses

Submucosal hemorrhages may be pinpoint size (petechiae) or larger (ecchymoses) (Figs. 3–40 and 3–41). This type of bleeding is generally seen intraorally because of either trauma or a blood dyscrasia. The palate, especially along the vibrating line at the junction of the hard and soft palates, is most commonly affected. Coughing, fellatio, and trauma from prosthetic appliances are etiologic factors.

Blood dyscrasias that may be associated with oral petechiae or ecchymoses include conditions such as leukemia, neutropenia, thrombocytopenia, hemophilia, and infectious mononucleosis.

Lesions appear red to blue to purple, depending on the age of the lesion. The lesions do not blanch on compression. Lesions for which there is no traumatic history should be regarded as possible oral expression of a blood dyscrasia.

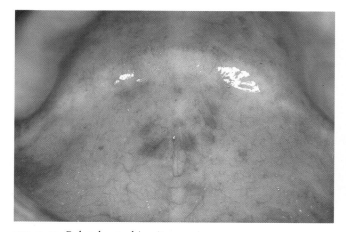

FIG. 3–40. Palatal petechiae (trauma)

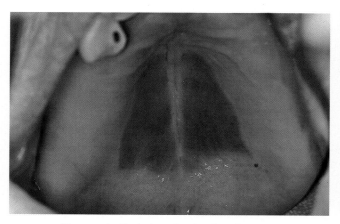

FIG. 3–41. Traumatically induced palatal ecchymoses

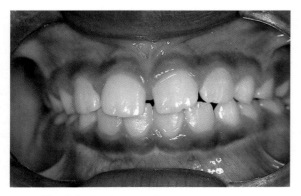

FIG. 3–42. Physiologic pigmentation

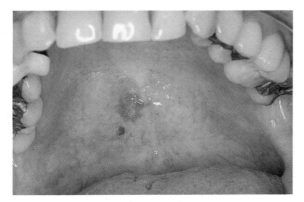

FIG. 3–43. Melanotic macule (postinflammatory)

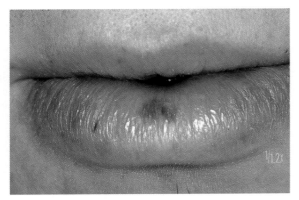

FIG. 3–44. Melanotic macules idiopathic

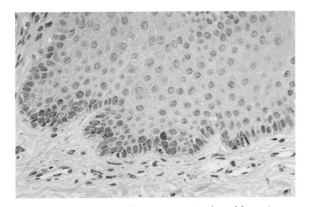

FIG. 3–45. Melanotic macule—pigment in basal keratinocytes

■ Physiologic Pigmentation

Physiologic pigmentation is symmetric and persistent, and does not change with time (Fig. 3–42). It does not mask gingival stippling or other architectural features of the mucosa. It most commonly affects the gingiva, although the tongue papillae and buccal mucosa may show patchy pigmentation. Microscopically, keratinocytes and subjacent macrophages contain melanin pigment. Melanocytes, found in the basal-epithelial zone, transfer mature pigmented melanosomes to surrounding keratinocytes.

■ Oral Melanotic Macule

The oral melanotic macule, or *focal melanosis*, is a pigmented lesion that may be an oral freckle, postinflammatory pigmentation (Fig. 3–43), or idiopathic (Fig. 3–44). It can also be associated with *Peutz-Jeghers syndrome* (perioral macules and intestinal polyposis) or *Addison's disease* (adrenal insufficiency). These lesions are commonly seen on the lips and gingiva, although any surface may be affected. Melanin pigment is found in basal keratinocytes and subjacent macrophages (Fig. 3–45). These lesions are of little significance, except to differentiate them from in situ melanoma and association with the two syndromes noted above.

■ Smoking-Associated Melanosis

Smoking, particularly cigarette smoking, may lead to melanin pigmentation of the gingiva and other mucosal sites (Fig. 3–46). This is seen predominantly in women, especially those taking birth control pills or hormonal eplacement therapy. The process is reversible and improves when the patient quits smoking. It is generally insignificant, except that it must be separated from other more serious pigmentary disorders, and it may be cosmetically objectionable.

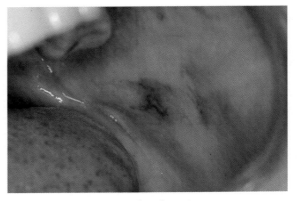

FIG. 3–46. Smoking-associated melanosis

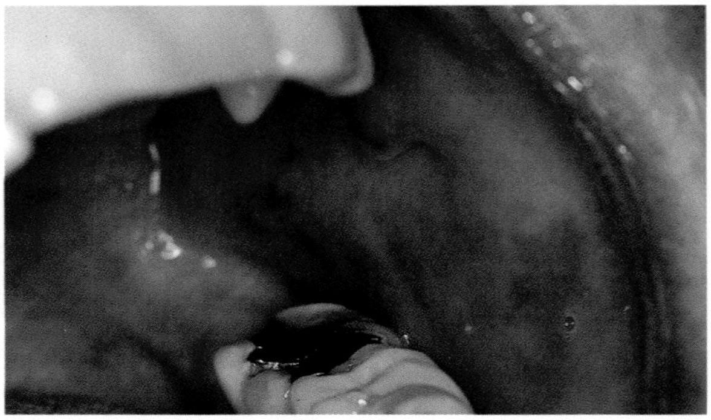

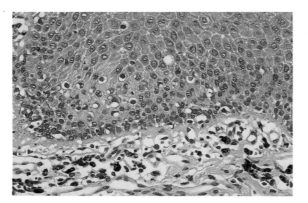

FIG. 3–47. Melanotic macules associated with Addison's disease

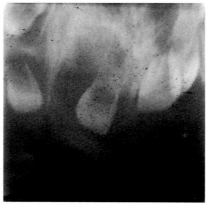

FIG. 3–48. Pigment distribution in Laugier-Hunzicker syndrome

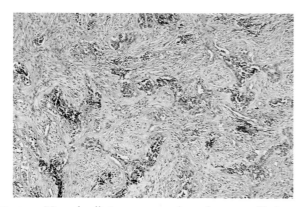

FIG. 3–49. Neuroectodermal tumor of infancy

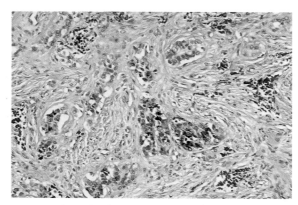

FIG. 3–50. Nested cells in neuroectodermal tumor of infancy

■ Peutz-Jeghers Syndrome

Perioral freckles or melanotic macules may suggest one of several syndromes. Peutz-Jeghers syndrome is an autosomal dominant condition in which patients develop perioral melanotic macules and intestinal polyposis. Melanin is seen in basal keratinocytes. The polyps are believed to be hamartomatous and have very limited neoplastic potential. They may, however, be responsible for abdominal pain, rectal bleeding, and diarrhea.

■ Addison's Disease

Addison's disease represents insufficiency of the adrenal cortex resulting from infection, autoimmune disease, or idiopathic causes. Reduced cortisol production leads to increased melanocyte-stimulating hormone production by the pituitary in a negative feedback relationship. This, along with increased ACTH production, results in stimulation of melanocytes and the production of excess pigment as melanotic macules (Fig. 3–47) or generalized darkening of the skin. Other signs and symptoms of this syndrome include weakness, weight loss, nausea, vomiting, and hypotension.

A third pigmentary syndrome or phenomenon known as *Laugier-Hunzicker* appears as melanotic macules of the oral mucous membrane (Fig. 3–48). This is an acquired disorder of unknown etiology and affects usually the lips, intraoral mucosa, and fingers. There is no known malignant potential of these pigmented patches.

■ Neuroectodermal Tumor of Infancy

This is a rare benign neoplasm of pigment-producing cells of neural crest origin. It typically occurs as a mass in the maxilla in infants usually less than 6 months of age. The lesion is darkly pigmented and presents as a poorly defined lucency of the anterior maxilla (Fig. 3–49). Microscopically, there are nests of small compact and medium-sized cells that contain melanin (Figs. 3–50 and 3–51). The lesion is excised, and recurrences are uncommon.

FIG. 3–51. High magnification of Figure 3–50 showing melanin

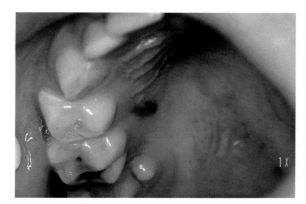

FIG. 3–52. Palatal nevus

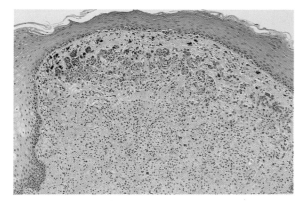

FIG. 3–53. Intramucosal nevus

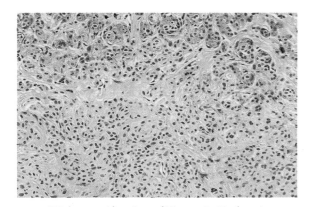

FIG. 3–54. High magnification of Figure 3–53 showing nests of nevus cells

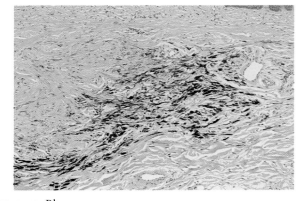

FIG. 3–55. Blue nevus

■ Melanocytic Nevi

The melanocytic or pigmented nevus is a collection of round or polygonal melanin pigment-producing cells that have migrated from the neural crests to sites in skin and rarely oral mucosa.

CLINICAL FEATURES
The nevus cells produce papules or nodules, most commonly in the palate (Fig. 3–52). Less frequently, the buccal mucosa, lips, gingiva, and alveolar ridge may be affected. The color is brown to black, and occasionally the same color as surrounding tissue due to low melanin production.

MICROSCOPIC FEATURES
Microscopically, nevus cells appear in a nested pattern, usually in the submucosa (intramucosal nevus) (Figs. 3–53 and 3–54). Rarely, nevus cells are found at the epithelial–connective tissue interface, in which case junctional nevus is the designation. This pattern is also seen in melanoma *in situ*; separation of these two lesions may be difficult. When nevus cells are found at both the epithelial–connective tissue interface and within submucosa, compound nevus is the designation used. A fourth type of nevus that is relatively common, especially in the palate, is known as *blue nevus*. This lesion is composed of deep-seated spindle-shaped melanin-producing cells (Figs. 3–55 and 3–56).

TREATMENT
Because early oral melanoma may simulate melanotic macule or junctional nevus, all pigmented lesions of undetermined diagnosis should be biopsied. Oral nevi probably have little or no capacity to undergo malignant transformation.

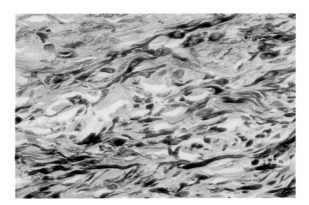

FIG. 3–56. High magnification of Figure 3–55 showing pigmented cells

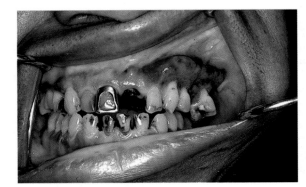

FIG. 3–57. Invasive melanoma

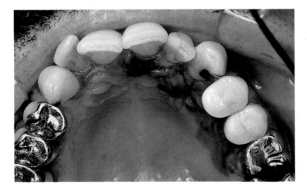

FIG. 3–58. *In situ* melanoma

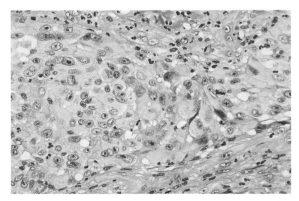

FIG. 3–59. Invasive oral amelanotic melanoma

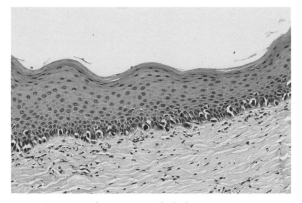

FIG. 3–60. *In situ* melanoma (epithelial–connective tissue interface)

■ Oral Melanoma

Oral melanomas are biologically aggressive and persistent neoplasms. Their clinical course is unpredictable, and outcome is characteristically fatal.

CLINICAL FEATURES

Oral melanomas are much less common than cutaneous melanomas. There are no known predisposing factors or geographic differences. Oral lesions usually occur after age 50 and are rarely seen before age 20. There is a very strong predilection for the palate and gingiva. Lesions are asymmetric and have irregular outlines. They also show variation in color from red to brown to black or blue. Occasionally they are multifocal, especially in the palate.

There appear to be two biologic subtypes of oral melanoma. One type shows an invasive or vertical growth pattern without significant lateral spread (Fig. 3–57). The other type of oral melanoma, called *in situ* melanoma, features a lateral growth phase lasting months to years followed by a vertical growth phase (Fig. 3–58). This may be confused with benign pigmentation.

MICROSCOPIC FEATURES

Invasive melanoma cells show atypical nuclear features and mitotic figures. Pigment is often but not always present (Fig. 3–59). For amelanotic melanomas, immunohistochemistry for melanoma-associated proteins (S-100, HMB45) must be done for confirmation. In cases of vertical invasion from an *in situ* melanoma, melanoma cells may appear spindled. This pattern is similar to *acral lentiginous melanoma* of the extremities. Neoplastic cells of *in situ* melanoma may show single or nested cells at the epithelial–connective tissue interface (Figs. 3–60 and 3–61). These cells may be well differentiated or may show considerable nuclear atypia. Intraepithelial spread is also sometimes seen. Any pigmentation with an interface or "junctional" pattern in a high-risk site (palate and gingiva) should be viewed with great suspicion as a possible *in situ* melanoma.

TREATMENT AND PROGNOSIS

The treatment of choice is surgery. Chemotherapy and radiotherapy may also be used, although a treatment record for these modalities has not been established. The prognosis for oral melanoma is generally very poor, with an overall 5-year survival rate of approximately 20%. Factors that contribute to this dismal outlook are tumor multifocality, tumor biology, and late stage of discovery and treatment.

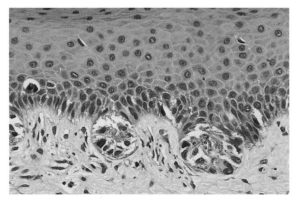

FIG. 3–61. *In situ* melanoma with interface tumor nests

CHAPTER 3: Red-Blue-Black Lesions ■ *Melanocytic Lesions*

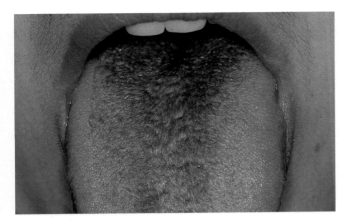

FIG. 3–62. Hairy tongue

■ Hairy Tongue

Hairy tongue is associated with one of many predisposing factors. The result is retention of keratin by the tongue papillae, giving the dorsum a "hairy" appearance (Fig. 3–62). The hyperkeratinized papillae may become colorized by exogenous factors such as coffee, tobacco, and/or chromogenic bacteria.

Factors contributing to this condition include antibiotic therapy, systemic corticosteroid use, radiation therapy, hydrogen peroxide rinses, and antacids. Other than being cosmetically objectionable, the lesion is of no significance. Treatment includes elimination of potential etiologic factors and improved oral hygiene, including tongue brushing. Podophyllum has also been used topically to reduce the lesion.

■ Amalgam Tattoo

Amalgam tattoo is an iatrogenic lesion that follows traumatic implantation of amalgam particles into mucous membrane. This may occur during amalgam restoration or fracture of an amalgam filling during extraction of a tooth. It is most frequently seen in the gingiva, buccal mucosa, tongue, and palate (Figs. 3–63 and 3–64). The lesions are slate-gray in color and do not change with time. Because amalgam is well tolerated by soft tissues, clinical signs of inflammation are usually not seen. If amalgam particles are sizeable, they may be detected in a soft tissue radiograph.

Microscopically, amalgam appears as black, finely divided particles found along collagen bundles and around blood vessels (Fig. 3–65). Occasionally a chronic inflammatory cell infiltrate is seen. Multinucleated foreign body giant cells may contain intracytoplasmic amalgam.

The significance of these lesions is that they must be separated from other more important pigmented lesions. If there is doubt about the clinical diagnosis, biopsy should be done.

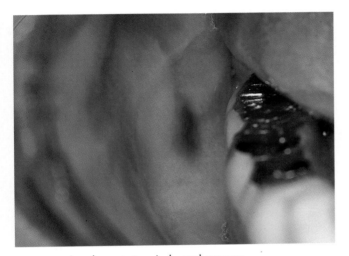

FIG. 3–63. Amalgam tattoo in buccal mucosa

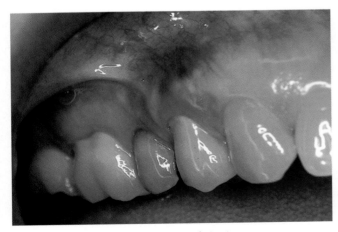

FIG. 3–64. Amalgam pigmentation of gingiva

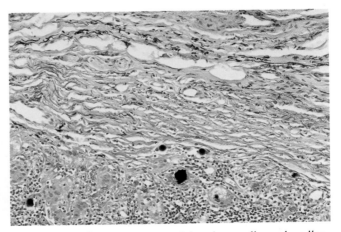

FIG. 3–65. Amalgam tattoo—particles along collagen bundles

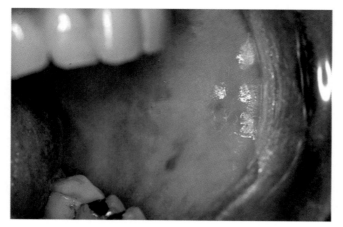
FIG. 3–66. Cyclophosphamide-induced pigmentation

■ Pigmentation Associated with Drugs

Some systemic drugs may stimulate melanocytes, or a form of the drug may become deposited in oral mucosa. These lesions appear as macular pigmentations ranging from brown to gray or black. Drugs known to induce mucosal pigmentation include minocycline, chloroquine, cyclophosphamide (Figs. 3–66 and 3–67), and zidovudine (Fig. 3–68). It is important to separate these pigmentary changes from melanoma.

Some heavy metals such as arsenic, bismuth, lead, and mercury may be responsible for oral pigmentation. Changes associated with these metals are usually due to occupational exposure to chemical vapors. Mucosa, especially gingiva, may appear gray to black in this situation. A pigmented line may be seen along the gingival margins due to reaction of the heavy metal with hydrogen sulfide in the gingival margin.

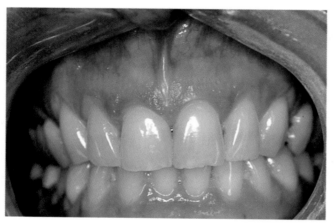
FIG. 3–67. Cyclophosphamide-induced pigmentation

■ Postinflammatory Pigmentation

This type of pigmentation is infrequently seen after a chronic inflammatory disease in the oral mucosa (Fig. 3–69). The buccal mucosa and tongue are the most commonly affected sites. This pigmentation can be classified as a type of oral melanotic macule. It is due to increased biologic activity of resident melanocytes; the numbers of melanocytes are not increased.

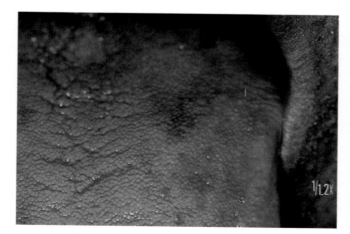
FIG. 3–68. Zidovudine-induced pigmentation of tongue

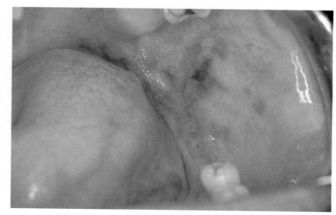
FIG. 3–69. Postinflammatory pigmentation in lichen planus

CHAPTER 3: Red-Blue-Black Lesions ■ *Other Pigmented Lesions*

CHAPTER 4

Papillary-Verrucal and Nodular Lesions

Verruciform

Squamous Papilloma and Oral Wart

Keratoacanthoma

Verrucous Carcinoma

Proliferative Verrucous Leukoplakia

Focal Epithelial Hyperplasia

Papillary Hyperplasia

Verruciform Xanthoma

Acanthosis Nigricans

Pyostomatitis Vegetans

Fibrous Lesions

Peripheral Fibroma

Gingival Cyst

Traumatic or Irritation Fibroma

Denture-Associated Hyperplasia

Generalized Gingival Hyperplasia

Nodular Fasciitis

Fibromatosis

Benign Fibrous Histiocytomas

Fibrosarcoma

Neural Lesions

Traumatic Neuroma

Neurilemmoma

Palisaded Encapsulated Neuroma

Neurofibroma

Mucosal Neuroma

Granular Cell Tumor

Congenital Gingival Granular Cell Tumor

Other Connective Tissue Lesions

Lymphangioma

Lipoma

Leiomyoma

Rhabdomyoma and Rhabdomyosarcoma

Lymphoma

Leukemia

Amyloidosis

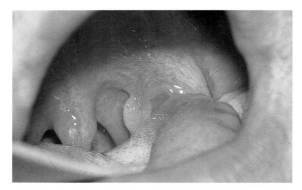

FIG. 4-1. Squamous papilloma adjacent to uvula

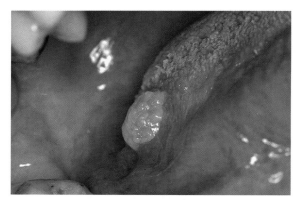

FIG. 4-2. Squamous papilloma, lateral tongue

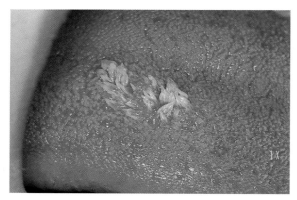

FIG. 4-3. Oral wart, dorsal tongue

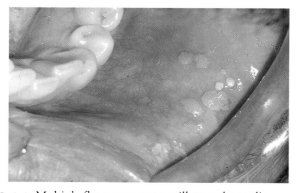

FIG. 4-4. Multiple flat squamous papillomas, lower lip

■ Squamous Papilloma and Oral Wart

Oral squamous papilloma is a generic term that indicates a focal papillary or verrucal growth of epithelium (with supporting connective tissue). Most are likely caused by human papillomavirus (HPV). When a lesion has the clinical/microscopic architecture of a common wart, the terms *verruca vulgaris* or *oral wart* can be used. When the epithelial growth does not exhibit the usual characteristics of verruca vulgaris, and HPV infection has not been proven, the generic *squamous papilloma* is preferred.

ETIOLOGY
Most oral squamous papillomas appear to be caused by HPV subtype 2, 6, 11, or 57. AIDS predisposes patients to multiple oral warts.

CLINICAL FEATURES
These lesions may be seen in any intraoral site (Figs. 4–1 through 4–4). There appears to be a slight predilection for the palate and uvula. The lesions present as either verruciform or cauliflower-like surface projections. The latter lesions usually are soft in texture.

Sexually transmitted warts (*condyloma acuminatum*) may be seen in intraoral sites (Fig. 4–5). These are caused by HPV subtypes 6 and 11. These lesions tend to be larger than papillomas and are broad-based.

MICROSCOPIC FEATURES
Papillary extensions of epithelium are supported by fibrovascular tissue (Figs. 4–6 through 4–8). In oral warts, koilocytosis (shrunken nucleus surrounded by a clear space) is seen in upper-level keratinocytes, suggesting HPV-induced changes. Also in warts, rete ridges at the periphery of the lesion point toward the center of the lesion.

Recently, *dysplastic warts* have been described in HIV-infected patients. They appear as small dome-shaped lesions with keratinocyte nuclear atypia and altered epithelial maturation (Figs. 4–9 and 4–10). A marked increase in cell cycle, as evidenced by immunohistochemical stain for proliferation-associated protein, is evident in these warts (Fig. 4–11). HPV common antigen is evident in upper-level keratinocyte nuclei (Fig. 4–12). Dysplastic warts in HIV-positive patients may be at risk for malignant transformation, although this has not been confirmed. At least some are associated with HPV subtypes 16 and 18.

TREATMENT
Surgical removal is the treatment of choice. Recurrences are uncommon, except for patients infected with HIV.

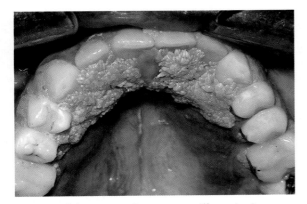

FIG. 4–5. Condyloma acuminatum, maxillary gingiva

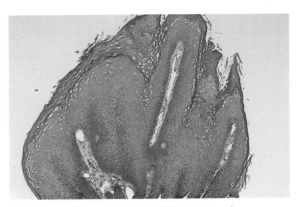

FIG. 4–6. Keratotic squamous papilloma or oral wart

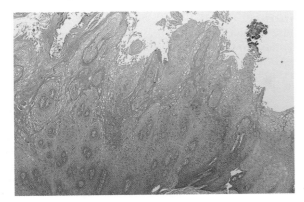

FIG. 4–7. Keratotic squamous papilloma or oral wart

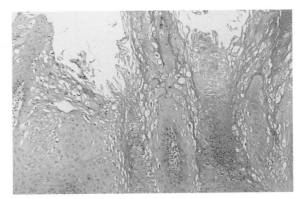

FIG. 4–8. High magnification of Figure 4–7 showing koilocytosis

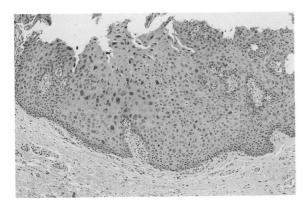

FIG. 4–9. Dysplastic wart in AIDS patient

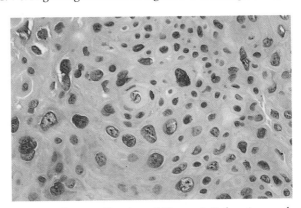

FIG. 4–10. High magnification of Figure 4–9 showing nuclear variation

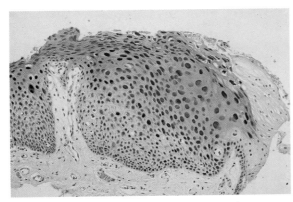

FIG. 4–11. Intense stain, dysplastic wart (cell cycle protein, PCNA)

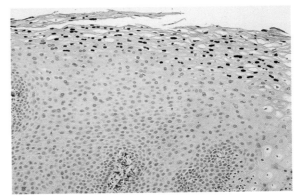

FIG. 4–12. Dysplastic wart, positive for HPV common antigen (top)

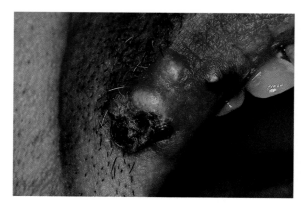

FIG. 4–13. Keratoacanthoma of upper lip

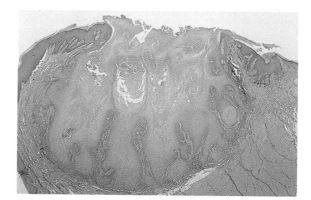

FIG. 4–14. Keratoacanthoma

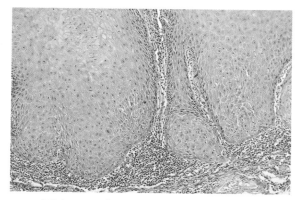

FIG. 4–15. High magnification of base of Figure 4–14

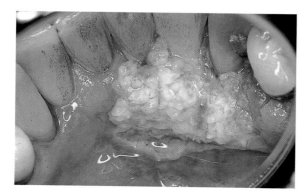

FIG. 4–16. Verrucous carcinoma of lingual gingiva

■ Keratoacanthoma

This is predominantly a skin lesion that rarely is seen on the lips or intraorally. It is a benign, self-limited lesion that mimics squamous cell carcinoma both clinically and microscopically.

Clinically, there is a central keratin plug and margins that are indurated (Fig. 4–13). After several weeks, the keratin is lost and the lesion begins to involute. The lesion will heal with scar.

Microscopically, the central keratin plug is surrounded by a "buttress" of normal epithelium (Figs. 4–14 and 4–15). The body of the lesion is composed of well-differentiated squamous cells that push into subjacent connective tissue.

TREATMENT
Because of their rarity intraorally and their similarity to squamous cell carcinoma, lesions suspected of being kera-toacanthoma must be biopsied. Some investigators believe that keratoacanthomas, in fact, represent very well-differentiated carcinomas.

■ Verrucous Carcinoma

This well-differentiated squamous cell carcinoma exhibits a verruciform profile (Fig. 4–16). Many of these lesions have been associated with the use of smokeless tobacco. Some develop in relation to proliferative verrucous leukoplakia.

The majority of intraoral verrucous carcinomas appear on the buccal mucosa and gingiva. Most are seen in males and in patients over age 50 years. The lesions are slow-growing and late to metastasize.

Microscopically, these well-differentiated lesions are often underdiagnosed as verrucous hyperplasia (Fig. 4–17). There is little or no significant cellular atypia. The growth pattern is both exophytic and endophytic. The lesion invades the submucosa as blunt ridges. The host response (inflammatory cell infiltrate) is variable.

TREATMENT
Surgery is generally used to treat these lesions. The role of radiation has not been fully explored, although recent reports suggest that it may be much more effective than previously appreciated. Lesions are more likely to recur locally than they are to metastasize.

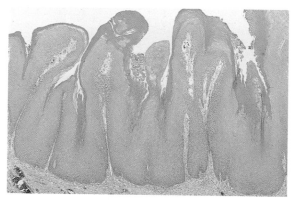

FIG. 4–17. Verrucous carcinoma

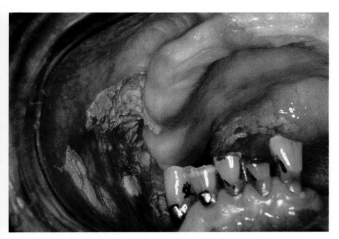

FIG. 4–18. Proliferative verrucous leukoplakia of buccal mucosa and palate

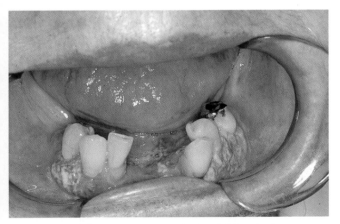

FIG. 4–19. Proliferative verrucous leukoplakia, gingiva

■ Proliferative Verrucous Leukoplakia

Proliferative verrucous leukoplakia is a clinical term used to describe a spectrum of change seen in some patients with multiple idiopathic white lesions. Lesions are initially flat and white due to excess keratin production. With time, lesions become elevated and frequently verruciform in profile (Figs. 4–18 and 4–19).

ETIOLOGY
Etiologic factors are not well understood, although a subset has been associated with human papillomavirus types 16 and 18. Smoking may contribute to the development of these lesions in some cases, but in many patients there is no smoking history. The disease may be particularly difficult to eradicate because of high recurrence potential. This is a notable problem when lesions affect the gingiva.

MICROSCOPIC FEATURES
Microscopically, proliferative verrucous leukoplakia encompasses lesions ranging from hyperkeratosis to invasive squamous cell carcinoma. The progression of this disease may take many years. Verrucous lesions tend to be underdiagnosed because they are remarkably well differentiated. Diagnosis is often made in retrospect after recurrence (Figs. 4–20 and 4–21). Lesions that become squamous cell carcinoma are usually well to moderately differentiated.

TREATMENT
The treatment of these lesions is predominantly surgical. The patient must also be committed to a lifetime of close follow-up care because of the multiplicity and the progressive nature of this phenomenon.

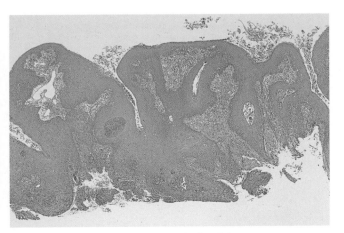

FIG. 4–20. Proliferative verrucous leukoplakia

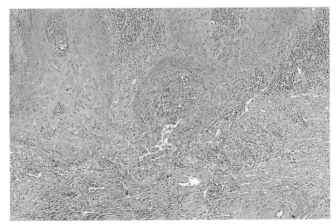

FIG. 4–21. High magnification of base of Figure 4–20

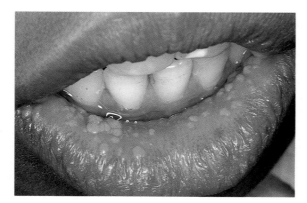

FIG. 4–22. Focal epithelial hyperplasia

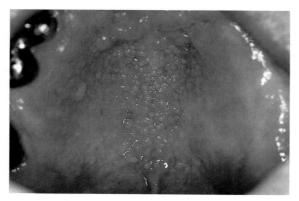

FIG. 4–23. Papillary hyperplasia

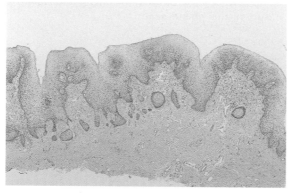

FIG. 4–24. Papillary hyperplasia

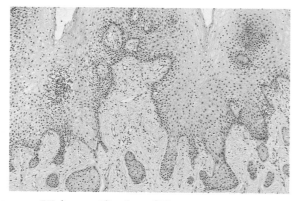

FIG. 4–25. High magnification of Figure 4–24

■ Focal Epithelial Hyperplasia

Also known as Heck's disease, this human papillomavirus-induced condition is seen predominantly in South and Central America.

Human papillomavirus subtypes 13 and 32 are believed to play an etiologic role in the development of this condition. Genetic factors may also be involved.

Focal epithelial hyperplasia presents as multiple nodular soft papules, usually on the buccal mucosa, lips, and tongue (Fig. 4–22). Papules are the same color as surrounding tissue and are painless.

Microscopically, the lesions show simple focal acanthosis and parakeratosis. Intracellular edema may also be present.

Differential diagnosis would include multiple verruca vulgaris, Cowden's syndrome (multiple hamartomas), Crohn's disease, and pyostomatitis vegetans. Clinicopathologic correlation is required for definitive diagnosis.

■ Papillary Hyperplasia

Papillary hyperplasia is a term used to describe one of the many reactive hyperplasias seen in oral mucous membranes. It most commonly occurs in the palate under an ill-fitting denture or partial denture, where it is also called *palatal papillomatosis*.

It is thought to be related to negative pressure, focally poor oral hygiene, and possibly overgrowth of *Candida albicans*.

Clinically, the mucosa exhibits a pebbly or cobblestone appearance (Fig. 4–23). The tissue is also usually red because of an inflammatory response with dilatation of capillaries.

Histologically, this lesion appears as numerous papillary projections covered by epithelium, often exhibiting pseudoepitheliomatous hyperplasia (Figs. 4–24 and 4–25). There is no dysplasia in these lesions, nor is there any risk for malignant transformation.

Treatment is related to the severity of the lesion and the condition of the denture. In mild cases, improved hygiene with antifungal therapy may be used, along with a relined denture. In more severe cases, surgical removal is necessary, with the construction of a new denture.

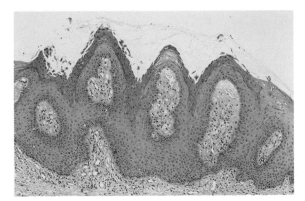

FIG. 4–26. Verruciform xanthoma

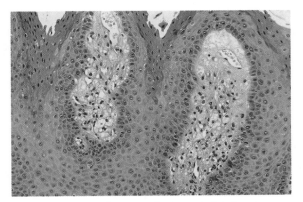

FIG. 4–27. High magnification of Figure 4–26 showing xanthoma cells

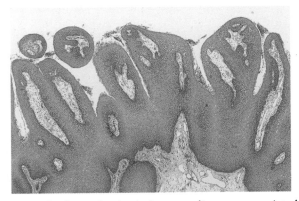

FIG. 4–28. Oral acanthosis nigricans, malignancy-associated

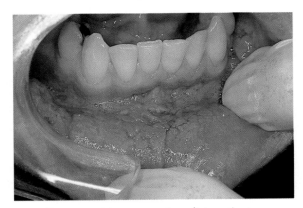

FIG. 4–29. Pyostomatitis vegetans in colitis patient

■ Verruciform Xanthoma

Verruciform xanthoma is an uncommon mucosal lesion that typically presents as a small papule (<1 cm in diameter) of the mucous membranes. The surface may be granular or papillary and white to red. Lesions are seen in adults, and the palate is often affected.

Microscopically, the lesion exhibits a warty surface architecture with numerous xanthoma cells (foamy macrophages) in the lamina propria (Figs. 4–26 and 4–27).

Other than differentiation from other papillary mucosal lesions, verruciform xanthoma is of little significance. The lesion does not recur after excision.

■ Acanthosis Nigricans

Acanthosis nigricans is predominantly a skin condition in which there are papillary plaques that are pigmented (melanin). These lesions are associated either with one of several benign systemic conditions or with the presence of an internal malignancy, usually intra-abdominal.

Oral lesions of acanthosis nigricans present as broad-based patches with a papillary architecture (Fig. 4–28). Oral lesions may be part of the so-called "malignant" acanthosis nigricans form.

■ Pyostomatitis Vegetans

Pyostomatitis vegetans, as part of a differential diagnosis for papillary lesions, represents mucosal expression of inflammatory bowel disease (e.g., ulcerative colitis, Crohn's disease). Lesions are yellow or light in color due to infiltration of the papillary epithelium by neutrophils and eosinophils (Figs. 4–29 and 4–30). Abscesses may develop within the lamina propria.

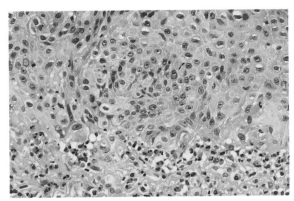

FIG. 4–30. Eosinophil infiltrate in subepithelium (patient in Figure 4–29)

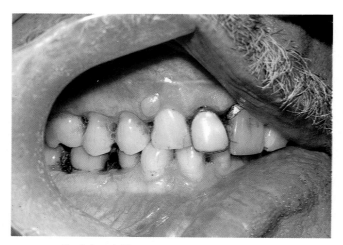

FIG. 4–31. Peripheral fibroma

■ Peripheral Fibroma

Peripheral fibroma is a focal reactive hyperplasia that occurs in the gingiva. It may arise from the gingival sulcus, interdental papilla, or attached gingiva. It is lighter than the surrounding tissue due to its relative avascularity (Figs. 4–31 and 4–32). The cause is thought to be chronic irritation, although a cause-and-effect relationship is often not apparent.

Microscopically, the bulk of the lesion is composed of hyperplastic fibrous tissue (Fig. 4–33). On occasion these lesions contain numerous multinucleated and stellate-shaped fibroblasts; this lesion has been called *giant cell fibroma* (Fig. 4–34). A subtype of peripheral fibroma is *peripheral ossifying fibroma*. This is a relatively cellular fibroblastic lesion with islands of new bone (Figs. 4–35 and 4–36).

These lesions are characteristically ulcerated. All types of peripheral fibromas are treated by excision to periosteum or periodontal ligament. Recurrences are occasionally associated with peripheral ossifying fibromas.

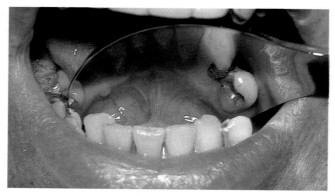

FIG. 4–32. Peripheral fibroma, lingual gingiva

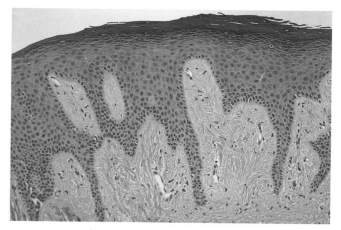

FIG. 4–33. Peripheral fibroma

■ Gingival Cyst

The gingival cyst presents as a nodular or elevated lesion of the gingiva. It is the same color as surrounding tissue or slightly bluish (Fig. 4–37). It is believed to result from the proliferation and cystic change of dental lamina rests that did not involute within the submucosa.

Microscopically, the cyst is lined by thin nonkeratinized epithelium with focal thickenings (Figs. 4–38 and 4–39). The microscopy is similar to that of a lateral periodontal cyst, suggesting a similar pathogenesis. Lesions are surgically removed with minimal risk of recurrence.

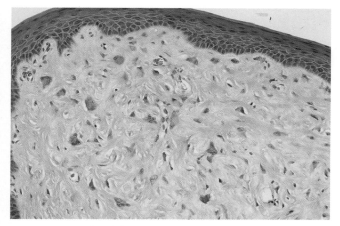

FIG. 4–34. Peripheral fibroma with stellate and giant cells

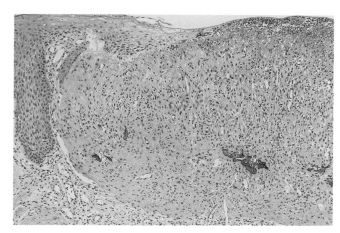

FIG. 4–35. Peripheral ossifying fibroma

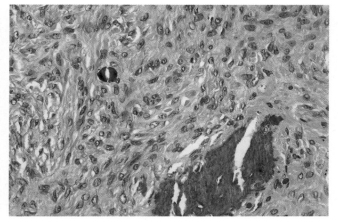

FIG. 4–36. High magnification of Figure 4–35 showing new bone

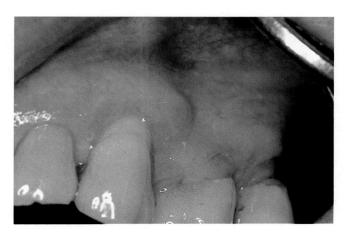

FIG. 4–37. Gingival cyst

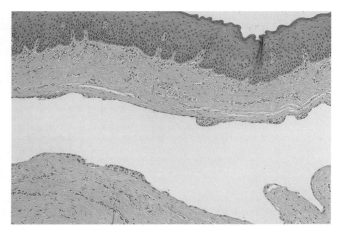

FIG. 4–38. Gingival cyst

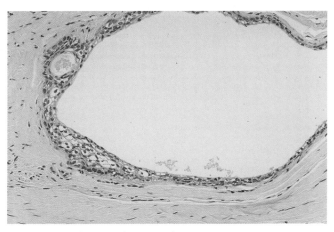

FIG. 4–39. High magnification of Figure 4–3

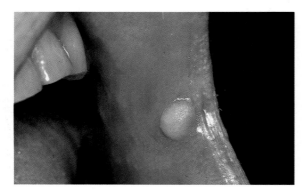

FIG. 4-40. Traumatic fibroma

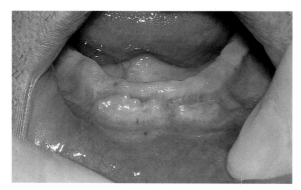

FIG. 4-41. Denture-associated hyperplasia

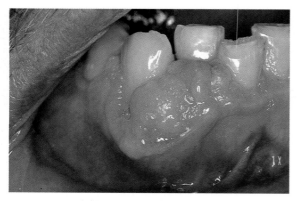

FIG. 4-42. Gingival fibrous hyperplasia, cyclosporine-related

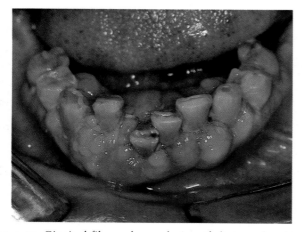

FIG. 4-43. Gingival fibrous hyperplasia, nifedipine-related

■ Traumatic or Irritation Fibroma

Traumatic or irritation fibroma is the term used to describe common focal fibrous hyperplasias (Fig. 4-40). By definition, these lesions are not gingival and are not associated with dentures; traditionally, the latter two lesions are designated peripheral fibroma and denture-associated hyperplasia, respectively. Traumatic fibromas occur in tissue that is most commonly traumatized, namely the buccal mucosa, lower lip, and lateral tongue surface.

■ Denture-Associated Hyperplasia

Denture-associated hyperplasia is related to chronic trauma from poorly fitting dentures (Fig. 4-41). As alveolar ridges become resorbed, the denture flange traumatizes the sulcular tissue. The result is the appearance of folds of hyperplastic scar, usually in the anterior maxillary and mandibular vestibules, where the results of denture trauma are most frequently seen.

■ Generalized Gingival Hyperplasia

Generalized gingival hyperplasia is associated with one of several factors. One is poor oral hygiene. This, especially in the presence of hormonal imbalance during puberty and pregnancy, can stimulate gingival fibroblasts. Another association is with drugs, such as phenytoin (Dilantin), cyclosporine (Fig. 4-42), and calcium channel blockers, such as nifedipine (Fig. 4-43). Leukemia, especially monocytic leukemia, may be associated with gingival enlargement due to either leukemic infiltrates or reactive hyperplasia associated with poor oral hygiene. There are also idiopathic forms of generalized gingival hyperplasia in which there is believed to be a hereditary predisposition or syndrome association. In all types of fibrous hyperplasia, well-collagenized and hyperplastic fibrous tissue characterizes these lesions. Epithelial hyperplasia and inflammation are variable (Fig. 4-44).

These fibrous hyperplasias are not hygienic or cosmetically acceptable. They are generally removed for diagnostic, esthetic, or functional purposes.

Clinically, these lesions all result in submucosal masses. Microscopically, they can exhibit overlapping features and are often considered together in a differential diagnosis.

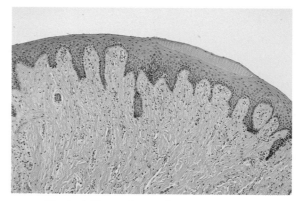

FIG. 4-44. Gingival fibrous hyperplasia

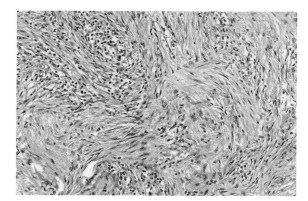
FIG. 4–45. Nodular fasciitis of buccal mucosa

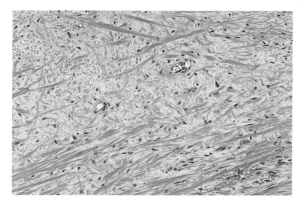
FIG. 4–46. Fibromatosis of floor of mouth

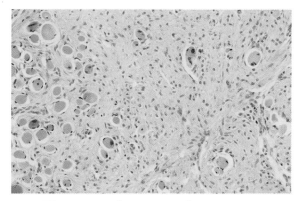
FIG. 4–47. Fibromatosis showing muscle invasion

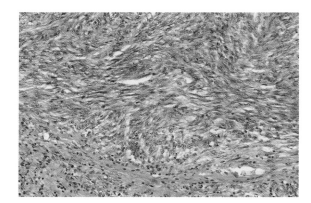
FIG. 4–48. Benign fibrous histiocytoma of tongue

■ Nodular Fasciitis

This is a reactive process that can be considered an inflammatory pseudotumor. The cause is unknown. It presents as a rapidly growing submucosal or subcutaneous mass that is occasionally painful. Approximately 10% of all cases are in the head and neck area. Microscopically, there is a proliferation of plump, well-differentiated fibroblasts (Fig. 4–45) which proliferate in an open pattern, frequently with myxoid areas. Mitotic figures may be abundant but are normal in appearance. Inflammatory cells and extravasated red cells are also part of the microscopic picture. The lesion is not encapsulated but is often circumscribed.

■ Fibromatosis

This is a benign but locally aggressive lesion noted for its recurrence potential, due in part to its infiltrative nature. The microscopy is deceptively bland, being composed of uniform compact fibroblasts surrounded by abundant collagen (Figs. 4–46 and 4–47). Nuclei are uniform, and mitotic figures are infrequently seen. Its bony counterpart is known as desmoplastic fibroma.

■ Benign Fibrous Histiocytoma

Benign fibrous histiocytoma is a proliferation of fibroblasts and presumably macrophages. It is unencapsulated but usually circumscribed. The lesion can be rather cellular, but the components are well differentiated (Fig. 4–48). Mitotic figures are infrequently seen and are normal. Recurrence is unlikely after surgical excision.

■ Fibrosarcoma

Oral *fibrosarcoma* is typically a well-differentiated malignancy. Spindle cells show nuclear atypia, and mitotic figures may be quite numerous (Fig. 4–49). A fascicular pattern is often seen, and the lesion is infiltrative. Separation from benign fibroblastic proliferations is often difficult. Recurrence, increasing cellularity with recurrence, and lack of inflammatory cell infiltrate would support a diagnosis of fibrosarcoma.

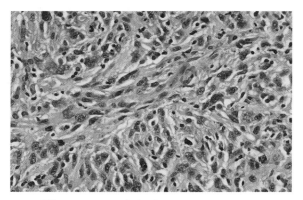
FIG. 4–49. Fibrosarcoma of gingiva

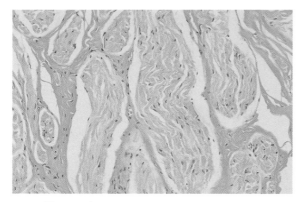

FIG. 4–50. Traumatic neuroma

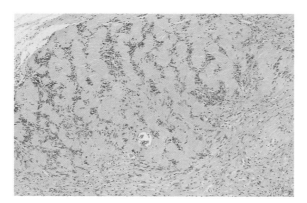

FIG. 4–51. Neurilemmoma

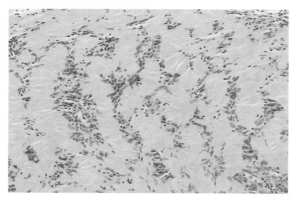

FIG. 4–52. High magnification of Figure 4–51

■ Traumatic Neuroma

This lesion represents an exuberant reparative response associated with damage to nerve tissue. It is seen in areas of nerve trauma and is commonly associated with extraction of a tooth, local anesthetic injection, or an accident (trauma). The lesion represents scar entwined with nerve tissue that has attempted to regenerate (Fig. 4–50). The resulting nodule of scar and nerve is painful on compression in about half of the cases. It usually does not recur after excision.

■ Neurilemmoma

Also known as *schwannoma*, this lesion is a benign neoplastic proliferation of Schwann cells. This asymptomatic submucosal mass may present at any age and in any oral location. It is usually solitary and occasionally occurs in bone. It is rarely associated with the syndrome neurofibromatosis.

Microscopically, neurilemmoma has a characteristic pattern of palisaded Schwann cell nuclei that surround acellular eosinophilic zones known as Verocay bodies (Figs. 4–51 and 4–52). These palisaded zones are sometimes known as Antoni A areas. When the cellular pattern is haphazard, the zone is known as Antoni B tissue.

■ Palisaded Encapsulated Neuroma

This is another benign neoplasm of Schwann cell origin. It exhibits a similar but slightly different microscopic pattern than neurilemmoma. It is more fascicular, with only a suggestion of nuclear palisading (Figs. 4–53 and 4–54). This lesion commonly presents as an asymptomatic nodule in the palate. It is usually solitary and is not syndrome-associated.

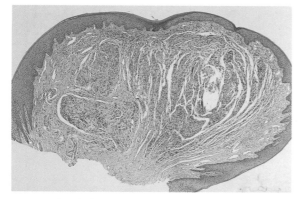

FIG. 4–53. Palisaded and encapsulated neuroma

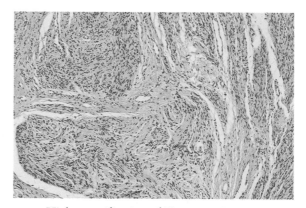

FIG. 4–54. High magnification of Figure 4–53

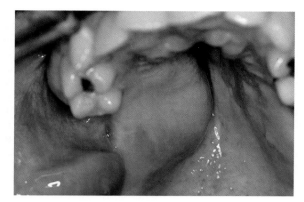

FIG. 4–55. Neurofibroma of palate

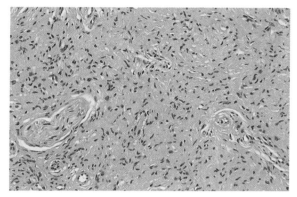

FIG. 4–56. Neurofibroma

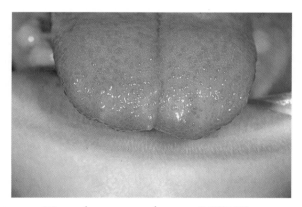

FIG. 4–57. Mucosal neuromas of tongue (MEN III)

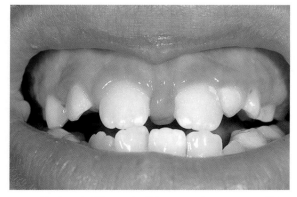

FIG. 4–58. Patient in Figure 4–57: mucosal neuromas, lip and gingiva

■ Neurofibroma

Neurofibromas may present as solitary or multiple nodules of Schwann cells or perineural fibroblasts. When multiple, they may represent part of the syndrome neurofibromatosis (von Recklinghausen's disease of skin). The syndrome is inherited as an autosomal dominant trait due to mutation of the NF1 or NF2 gene.

Lesions present as uninflamed asymptomatic submucosal masses. These lesions are soft and may be discrete nodules or diffuse masses (Fig. 4–55). The tongue, buccal mucosa, and vestibule are most commonly affected. In addition to multiple lesions, neurofibromatosis includes café au lait macules of the skin, bone lesions, and neurologic abnormalities. The neurofibromas of this syndrome are at risk for malignant change (5% to 15% of patients).

Microscopically, lesions are composed of spindle-shaped cells, often with wavy nuclei (Fig. 4–56). The matrix holding these cells is delicate and fibrillar ("neuroid"). Lesions may be well circumscribed or blend into surrounding connective tissue. Mast cells are typically scattered throughout these lesions.

■ Mucosal Neuroma

Mucosal neuromas are part of the multiple endocrine neoplasia syndrome type III (MEN III). This autosomal dominant disease also includes medullary carcinoma of the thyroid, pheochromocytoma of the adrenal, characteristic facies, and occasionally café au lait macules. Mucosal neuromas are characteristically seen on the tongue, lips, and buccal mucosa (Figs. 4–57 and 4–58). They are usually less than 1 cm in diameter, asymptomatic, and soft. Oral lesions may be the first apparent sign of this syndrome.

Microscopically, mucosal neuromas are composed of serpiginous bands of delicate nerve tissue (Fig. 4–59). Axons can be found in the nerve bundles.

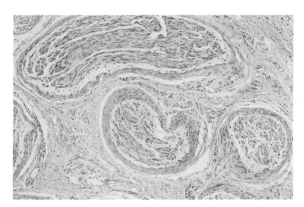

FIG. 4–59. Mucosal neuroma of MEN III

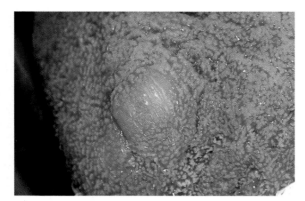

FIG. 4–60. Granular cell tumor of tongue

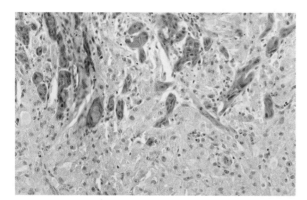

FIG. 4–61. Granular cell tumor and pseudoepitheliomatous hyperplasia

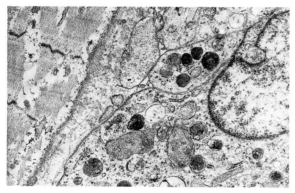

FIG. 4–62. Autophagic vacuoles in granular cell (muscle, left)

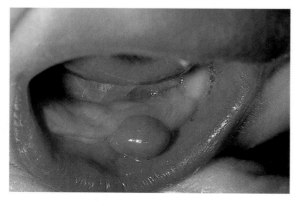

FIG. 4–63. Congenital gingival granular cell tumor

Granular Cell Tumor

This lesion, believed to be of neural origin, presents as a submucosal mass, typically in the tongue. It is benign, has no malignant potential, and rarely recurs after simple excision.

Once thought to originate from skeletal muscle, the lesion was known as granular cell myoblastoma. However, because of ultrastructural and immunohistochemical evidence, the unusual granular cells that make up this lesion appear to be of neural, probably Schwann cell, origin. Tumor cells are positive for S-100, CEA, CD57, CD68, and collagen IV. Granular cell tumors, also found in other sites, such as the skin, gastrointestinal tract, and respiratory tract, are microscopically similar.

Clinically, oral granular cell tumors may occur at any age, and females seem to be affected more commonly than males. The tongue is the favored site (Fig. 4–60). Granular cell tumor presents as an uninflamed asymptomatic mass less than 2 cm in diameter. The overlying epithelium is intact. Multiple tongue lesions have been described.

Microscopically, the characteristic granular cells exhibit a flocculent or granular cytoplasm with a small, usually centrally placed, vesicular nucleus. Ultrastructurally, the cells are filled with autophagic vacuoles (Fig. 4–62). Of note is the epithelial hyperplasia that often overlies these tumors (Fig. 4–61). This pseudoepitheliomatous pattern has occasionally been mistaken for squamous cell carcinoma, although there is no inflammatory infiltrate that is characteristically seen in oral cancers.

Congenital Gingival Granular Cell Tumor

Also known as *congenital epulis*, this is another tumescence composed of granular cells. It occurs on the alveolar ridge of infants and is usually pedunculated (Fig. 4–63). It is surgically removed and does not recur.

The congenital epulis, like the granular cell tumor, contains cells with flocculent or granular cytoplasm (Fig. 4–64). It is ultrastructurally and immunohistochemically similar but not identical to granular cell tumor. Some features suggest a possible origin from smooth muscle. Pseudoepitheliomatous hyperplasia is not seen in association with the congenital epulis.

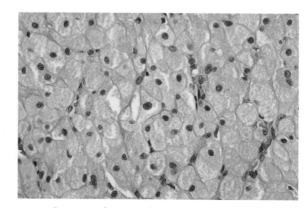

FIG. 4–64. Congenital gingival granular cell tumor

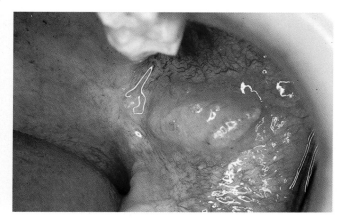

FIG. 4–65. Lymphangioma of buccal mucosa

■ Lymphangioma

CLINICAL FEATURES

Lymphangioma presents as a painless nodular swelling in which there are vesicle-like areas that represent superficially located lymphatic vessels. The color is usually lighter than the surrounding tissue, although mixed lymphangioma-hemangiomas may occur, resulting in red or even purple discoloration (Figs. 4–65 and 4–66). The lesions are crepitant on palpation.

Intraorally, the tongue is the most commonly affected site. Lymphangiomas seen in the neck of infants are known as *cystic hygroma* or *hygroma colli*. The neck lesions can be remarkably large and may lead to respiratory distress because of their location.

HISTOPATHOLOGY

Abundant numbers of endothelium-lined lymphatic channels expand the submucosa (Fig. 4–67). Vessels characteristically abut the basement membrane of the overlying epithelium (Fig. 4–68). The lymphatic vessels blend into the surrounding soft tissue without circumscription or encapsulation.

TREATMENT

Surgical removal is the treatment of choice. Staged surgical procedures may be needed for large lesions. Recurrence is common due to the lack of circumscription of this lesion.

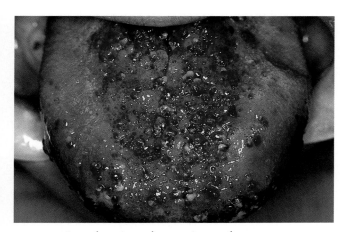

FIG. 4–66. Lymphangioma-hemangioma of tongue

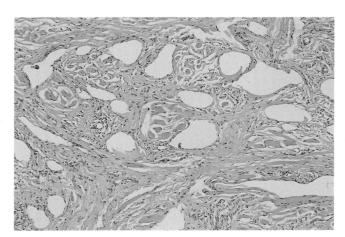

FIG. 4–67. Lymphangioma in deep submucosa

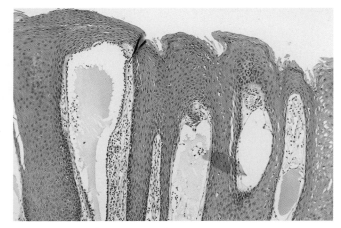

FIG. 4–68. Lymphangioma in lamina propria

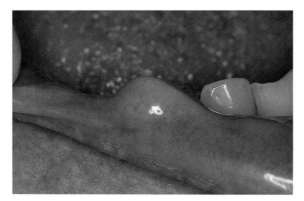

FIG. 4–69. Lipoma of lip

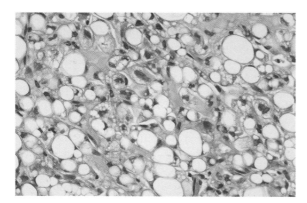

FIG. 4–70. Liposarcoma

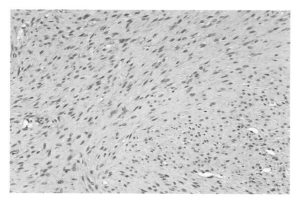

FIG. 4–71. Leiomyoma

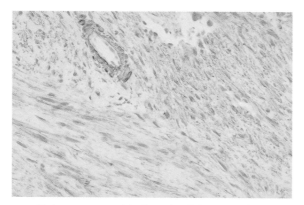

FIG. 4–72. Leiomyoma positively stained for smooth muscle actin

■ Lipoma

Lipoma is an uncommon benign neoplasm of the oral mucosa. It has been described in all locations, although the buccal mucosa and lip seem to be favored (Fig. 4–69). The lesion presents as a yellowish submucosal mass with intact overlying epithelium. Microscopically, the tumors consist of a lobular proliferation of mature fat that is typically well circumscribed if not encapsulated.

The malignant counterpart, liposarcoma, is rarely seen in oral mucosa. When present, it develops as a relatively slow-growing mass. Microscopically, several subtypes have been described. Common to all of them are tumor cells with atypical nuclei and cytoplasmic vacuoles (fat) of varying size and shape (Fig. 4–70). Surgery and radiation are used to ablate these lesions.

■ Leiomyoma

This benign smooth muscle neoplasm is relatively uncommon in the oral mucosa. Like other benign neoplasms, it presents as a slow-growing, asymptomatic submucosal mass with intact overlying epithelium. Microscopy shows a cellular spindled proliferation with many prominent small capillaries (Fig. 4–71). Immunohistochemistry can be used to demonstrate muscle protein (smooth muscle actin) in these cells (Fig. 4–72). A microscopic subtype known as *vascular leiomyoma*, which has numerous thick-walled vessels in association with the spindle cells, is occasionally seen in the oral mucosa (Fig. 4–73).

Leiomyosarcoma is rarely seen in the oral mucosa. This spindle-cell malignancy shows nuclear atypia and immunohistochemical evidence of smooth muscle protein.

Neoplasms of skeletal muscle origin are rare but appear to have a predilection for head and neck soft tissues.

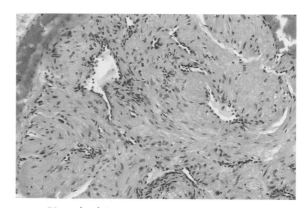

FIG. 4–73. Vascular leiomyoma

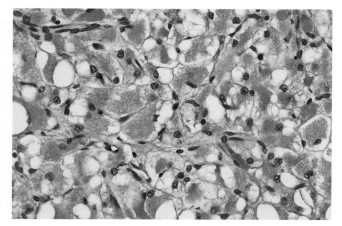

FIG. 4–74. Rhabdomyoma

■ Rhabdomyoma

Rhabdomyoma may be seen at any age, although middle age is the typical time of presentation. The tongue, floor of the mouth, soft palate, and buccal mucosa are the sites most frequently affected.

The microscopy of rhabdomyoma mimics the microscopy of skeletal muscle (Fig. 4–74). A circumscribed mass of well-differentiated cells with bright-pink cytoplasm is characteristic. Cross-striations can often be seen in the tumor cells. Lesions are excised and generally do not recur.

■ Rhabdomyosarcoma

Rhabdomyosarcomas occur in the head and neck in one of three histologic subtypes: pleomorphic, embryonal, or alveolar. The pleomorphic type is relatively well differentiated and is composed of strap and spindle cells that rarely show cross-striations (Fig. 4–75). Nuclei can be remarkably atypical and bizarre. The embryonal type is composed of small round cells in which there is minimal cytoplasm (Figs. 4–76 and 4–77). Embryonal rhabdomyosarcoma is often included in the microscopic differential of other head and neck round cell tumors (e.g., lymphoma, melanoma, olfactory neuroblastoma). The third alveolar variant of this malignancy is very rarely seen. It appears as a compartmentalized or alveolar proliferation of compact cells with small amounts of cytoplasm.

Rhabdomyosarcoma in the head and neck is characteristically seen in children. It presents as a rapidly growing mass of usually the tongue or soft palate. A combination of surgery, radiation, and chemotherapy is now used to treat patients with this aggressive malignancy. Survival rates have improved significantly with this multimodal therapy to better than 70%.

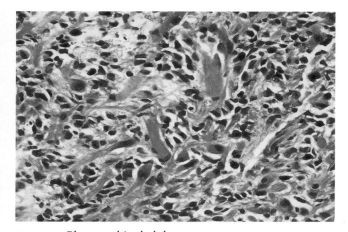

FIG. 4–75. Pleomorphic rhabdomyosarcoma

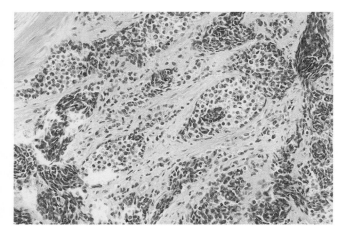

FIG. 4–76. Embryonal rhabdomyosarcoma

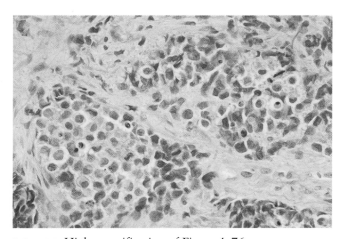

FIG. 4–77. High magnification of Figure 4–76

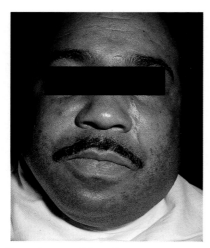

FIG. 4–78. Bilateral cervical lymphoma

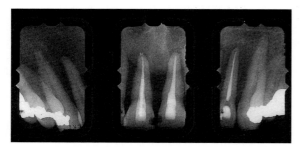

FIG. 4–79. Lymphoma in anterior maxilla

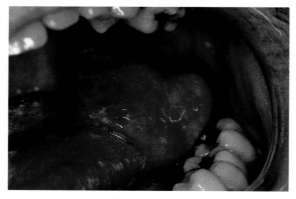

FIG. 4–80. HIV-associated oral lymphoma

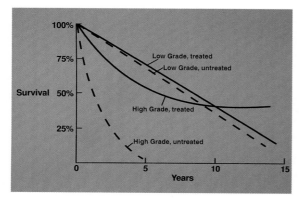

FIG. 4–81. Survival curves for lymphomas (modified from Grogan et al. Hematol Oncol Clin N Am 11:819–842, 1997)

■ Lymphoma

Malignancies of lymphoid cells (Hodgkin's and non-Hodgkin's lymphomas) are relatively common neoplasms of lymph nodes in the head and neck (Fig. 4–78). Extranodal oral lymphomas, presenting as either primary or secondary disease, are relatively uncommon (Fig. 4–79). Recently, with the emergence of HIV infection, the frequency of oral lymphomas has increased (Fig. 4–80). Hodgkin's lymphoma rarely involves the oral cavity and is excluded from this discussion.

Middle-aged and elderly patients are most commonly affected by oral lymphoma, except for Burkitt's lymphoma, which is often seen in children. When occurring in lymphoid tissue, a mass is seen in Waldeyer's ring. Extranodal disease typically appears in the palate as a smooth surfaced or ulcerated mass. Other soft tissue sites may be affected as well. Not uncommonly, lymphoma presents as a bony lesion, where it causes a radiolucency and elicits the symptoms of pain and paresthesia. Oral lymphomas may present before, concomitantly with, or after lymph node expression.

Microscopically, lymphomas represent uncontrolled proliferation of lymphoid cells that can be classified into one of several cell types. These classifications take into consideration the size of the neoplastic cells, their maturation and differentiation, and the microscopic pattern. These features taken together have been useful in predicting behavior and outcome. Several classification schemes have been devised for lymphomas. The Working Formulation, the Revised European-American Lymphoma classification (REAL), and the Kiel classifications are in relatively common use.

Oral lymphomas from HIV-negative patients are typically of the diffuse type. They are composed of moderately to well-differentiated small and large lymphoid cells (Figs. 4–82 and 4–83). These are generally low- to intermediate-grade lesions. In HIV-infected patients, a distinct shift to predominantly high-grade tumors is seen (Fig. 4–84). Cells are generally larger and poorly differentiated, with Epstein-Barr virus frequently present in the cells (Fig. 4–85). Oral lymphomas from both HIV-positive and HIV-negative populations are almost always of the B-cell type.

Treatment of lymphoma depends on the clinical extent or stage of the disease. Generally, radiation therapy is used for localized disease. Chemotherapy or combination chemotherapy and radiation is used for more extensive disease. Because some low-grade tumors have a protracted course and respond very poorly to therapy, no treatment may be elected for patients with these lesions (Fig. 4–81). AIDS-associated lymphomas are associated with a relatively poor prognosis.

■ Leukemia

Leukemias, especially monocytic leukemia, may express themselves in the mouth at some time during the course of the disease. Infiltrates may be seen in bone, causing lucencies with pain and paresthesia, or they may be seen in the gingiva, producing generalized gingival enlargement (Figs. 4–86 and 4–87). Oral leukemia-associated lesions characteristically appear after systemic disease has been identified.

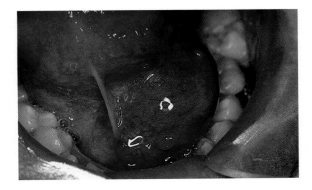

FIG. 5–6. Mucus retention cyst (ranula), floor of mouth

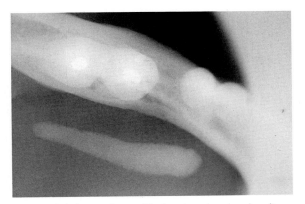

FIG. 5–7. Sialolith in submandibular duct (occlusal radiogram)

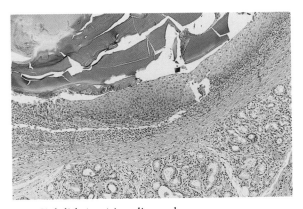

FIG. 5–8. Sialolith (top) in salivary duct

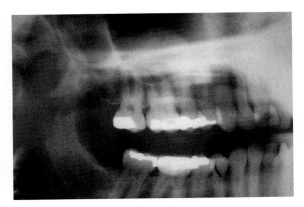

FIG. 5–9. Antral or maxillary sinus retention cyst

■ Mucus Retention Cyst

This lesion results from obstruction of a salivary gland duct. Retained mucin is surrounded by stretched ductal epithelium, giving the lesion a pseudocystic appearance microscopically.

ETIOLOGY AND PATHOGENESIS

Mucus retention cyst results from a duct blockage due to inspissated mucin, sialolith, periductal scar, or compression by neoplasm adjacent to the duct. Sialoliths represent precipitation of calcium carbonate and calcium phosphate in a central nidus of cellular debris and mucin. Sialolithiasis is most commonly seen in the floor of the mouth, although it may occur in any region where salivary gland tissue is found.

CLINICAL FEATURES

Mucus retention cyst is most commonly seen in the floor of the mouth, where it characteristically causes a large bluish dome-shaped swelling known as *ranula* (Fig. 5–6). Ranula is a clinical term that also includes mucus extravasation phenomenon in this site. Mucus retention cyst, when occurring in minor salivary gland, is usually seen in the upper lip, followed by palate, buccal mucosa, and floor of the mouth. Lesions are typically asymptomatic and result in a submucosal swelling that is often bluish.

MICROSCOPIC FEATURES

The salivary gland excretory duct is markedly dilated and contains inspissated mucin or a calcified sialolith (Figs. 5–7 and 5–8). The retained mucin is surrounded by thinned ductal epithelium. Unless there is some escape of mucin through the duct wall, there is a minimal inflammatory cell infiltrate.

TREATMENT

Mucus retention cyst of the minor salivary gland requires removal of the obstruction as well as the associated gland. For sialolithiasis of major salivary glands, removal of a stone can sometimes be accomplished without extirpation of the associated gland. This depends on the location of the stone (execretory duct or smaller intralobular duct(s)), and the number and size of stones.

■ Antral or Maxillary Sinus Retention Cyst

This is a common finding on panoramic radiographs and is of little or no clinical significance (Fig. 5–9). It represents blockage of a sinus salivary gland duct. Most lesions are asymptomatic and require no treatment. Lesions are usually diagnostic radiographically and appear as a homogeneous, slightly opaque, dome-shaped lesion on the floor of the maxillary sinus.

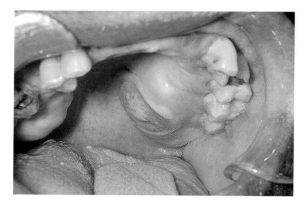

FIG. 5–10. Mixed tumor of palate

■ Mixed Tumor

Benign salivary gland tumors present typically as submucosal masses (Fig. 5–10). Lesions are asymptomatic and slow-growing. These benign tumors can appear in any site, although the palate is favored by mixed tumor and the upper lip by monomorphic adenoma. They may be seen at any age, but are typically found in adults. Mixed tumors occasionally recur, presumably due to tumor extension beyond a pseudocapsule. This appears to be of greater significance in major glands than minor glands.

Microscopically, mixed tumors are composed of a mixture of neoplastic epithelium and mesenchyme (Figs. 5–11 and 5–12). The epithelial component typically makes pseudoducts as well as networks and sheets of cohesive cells. The mesenchymal component is remarkably variable, ranging from myxoid connective tissue to hyalinized connective tissue to cartilage or bone (Fig. 5–13). Of diagnostic significance is the finding of plasmacytoid cells (myoepithelial cells) (Fig. 5–14).

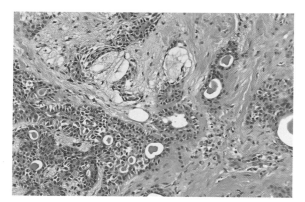

FIG. 5–11. Mixed tumor

■ Monomorphic Adenoma

Monomorphic adenomas are composed of a single epithelial cell type with minimal amounts of supporting connective tissue. There are a number of patterns or subtypes, mostly of academic interest, which are known as canalicular, tubular, trabecular, or basaloid (Figs. 5–15 through 5–19). Monomorphic adenomas composed of all plasmacytoid or spindle-shaped cells are called myoepitheliomas (Fig. 5–20).

■ Intraductal Papilloma

Minor salivary glands are host to several intraductal papillomas. One, known as *inverted ductal papilloma*, is a characteristic intraductal lobular proliferation lined by columnar cells interspersed with goblet cells (Fig. 5–21). Another papilloma, known as *sialadenoma papilliferum*, presents as a superficial papillary lesion connected directly to the surface (Fig. 5–22). Papillary projections are lined by columnar and thin stratified squamous epithelium. Finally, a simple branching *intraductal papilloma* has been described within the excretory ductal system.

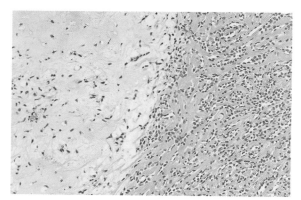

FIG. 5–12. Mixed tumor

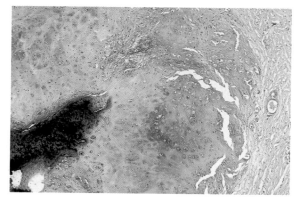

FIG. 5–13. Mixed tumor with focal bone differentiation

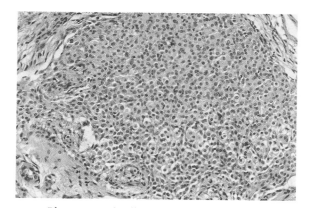

FIG. 5–14. Plasmacytoid cells in a mixed tumor

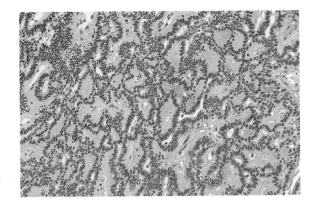

FIG. 5-15. Monomorphic adenoma, canalicular type

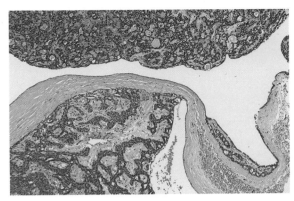

FIG. 5-16. Multifocal canalicular adenoma

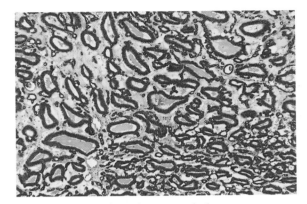

FIG. 5-17. Monomorphic adenoma, tubular type

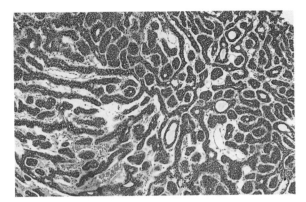

FIG. 5-18. Monomorphic adenoma, trabecular type

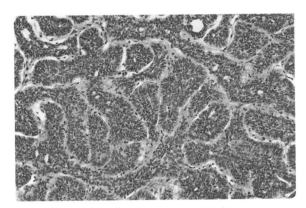

FIG. 5-19. Monomorphic adenoma, basaloid type

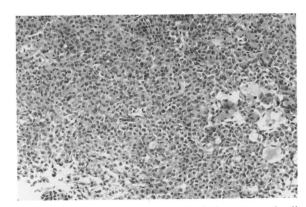

FIG. 5-20. Myoepithelioma composed of plasmacytoid cells

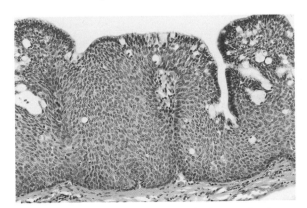

FIG. 5-21. Inverted ductal papilloma of salivary gland

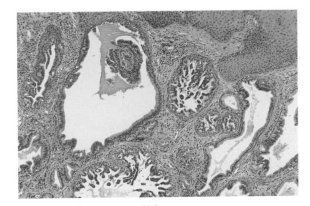

FIG. 5-22. Sialadenoma papilliferum

CHAPTER 5: Salivary Gland Lesions ■ *Adenomas*

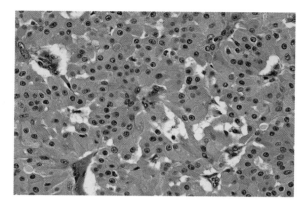

FIG. 5–23. Oncocytoma

■ Oncocytoma

Oncocytoma is a rare salivary gland tumor seen usually in the parotid. Occasionally oral lesions are found, particularly in the palate. Microscopically, oncocytoma is composed of a well-encapsulated mass of uniform cells with bright-pink cytoplasm (Fig. 5–23). The nucleus is usually centrally placed. Occasionally, due probably to fixation artifact, oncocytomas appear as clear cell tumors (Fig. 5–24). Ultrastructurally, oncocytomas contain abundant amounts of mitochondria (Fig. 5–25). There is a very rare malignant counterpart (*malignant oncocytoma*) in which cells show cytologic atypia and an invasive pattern.

■ Warthin's Tumor

Warthin's tumor, also known as *papillary cystadenoma lymphomatosum*, is an uncommon lesion seen predominantly in the parotid. It is occasionally bilateral, and when found in the tail of the parotid may mimic other neoplasms of the submandibular space. Warthin's tumor rarely arises within minor salivary glands. Microscopically, there is an epithelial component composed of a bilayer of oncocytes in a papillary configuration, and there is a lymphoid component in which mature lymphocytes with germinal centers are seen supporting the oncocytes (Figs. 5–26 and 5–27). The reason for the pink cytoplasm of the oncocytes is related to protein staining of the abundant mitochondria.

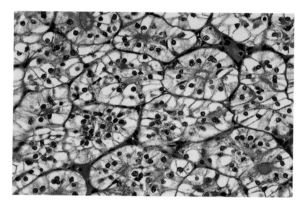

FIG. 5–24. Oncocytoma with clear cell change

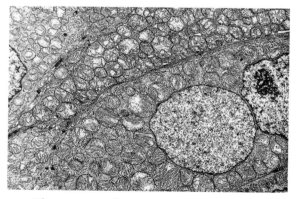

FIG. 5–25. Ultrastructure of oncocytoma showing mitochondria

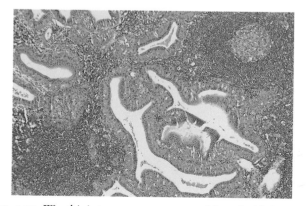

FIG. 5–26. Warthin's tumor: oncocytes and lymphoid tissue

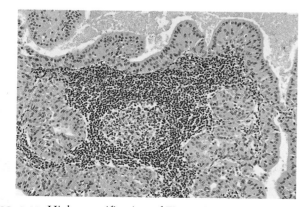

FIG. 5–27. High magnification of Figure 5–26

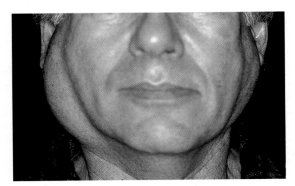

FIG. 5–28. Bilateral parotid swelling of Sjögren's syndrome

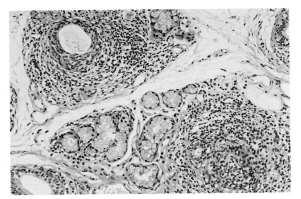

FIG. 5–29. Lymphocytic foci in salivary gland biopsy

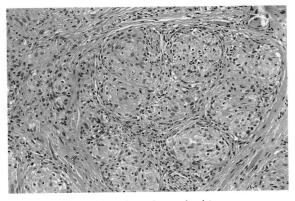

FIG. 5–30. Granuloma from lower lip biopsy

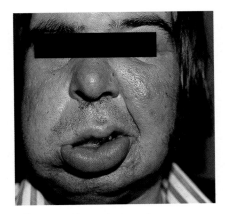

FIG. 5–31. Melkersson-Rosenthal syndrome

■ Sjögren's Syndrome

This is a chronic autoimmune disease in which lymphocytes infiltrate and replace parenchyma of salivary glands, lacrimal glands, and other exocrine glands. This eventually results in dry mouth (xerostomia) and dry eyes (keratoconjunctivitis sicca). When these tissues alone are affected, the condition is known as primary Sjögren's syndrome. If the patient also has another autoimmune disease, such as rheumatoid arthritis, the condition is known as secondary Sjögren's syndrome. The cause or trigger of this phenomenon is unknown. However, viruses (especially retrovirus, Epstein-Barr virus, and other herpesviruses) have been suspected as having an etiologic role.

This is a disease of older adults and especially women. In addition to dry mouth and eyes, patients may show bilateral soft parotid swelling (up to 50% of patients) (Fig. 5–28). With dry mouth, patients are predisposed to dental caries, candidiasis, and sensitive mucosa.

DIAGNOSIS
Diagnosis is based on history, physical examination, laboratory studies, and tissue biopsy. Decreased lacrimal secretion can be detected by the Schirmer test. Salivary involvement can be assessed through one of several tests, the best being biopsy of lower lip minor salivary glands. These glands reflect the changes seen in major salivary glands and lacrimal glands. Aggregates of lymphocytes are distributed throughout glandular tissue without other physical signs of inflammatory disease (Fig. 5–29). These foci of 50 or more lymphocytes are found typically directly adjacent to intact acinar structures. It has been determined that if there is more than one lymphocytic focus per 4 mm^2 of glandular tissue, the tissue change is consistent with the salivary component of Sjögren's syndrome. Significant laboratory findings would include identification of autoantibodies (rheumatoid factor, antinuclear antibodies, and Sjögren's syndrome-associated antibodies SS-A and SS-B). Coexisting rheumatoid arthritis or other systemic autoimmune disease would be necessary to make the diagnosis of secondary Sjögren's syndrome.

TREATMENT
Treatment is essentially symptomatic. It is important for patients to have excellent oral hygiene to combat the effects of xerostomia. Patients are at risk for malignant transformation of their disease to lymphoma.

■ Granulomatous Cheilitis

Granulomatous cheilitis is a diagnosis made after exclusion of other granulomatous diseases such as sarcoidosis, tuberculosis, and Crohn's disease. Granulomatous cheilitis presents as a swollen lip that, when biopsied, shows numerous noncaseating granulomas (Fig. 5–30). When seen in company with fissured tongue and facial paralysis, the condition is known as *Melkersson-Rosenthal syndrome* (Fig. 5–31). The cause of granulomatous cheilitis is unknown, making treatment empirical. Control, however, has been achieved to some degree with intralesional injection of corticosteroids.

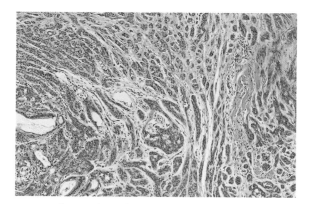

FIG. 5-32. Polymorphous low-grade adenocarcinoma

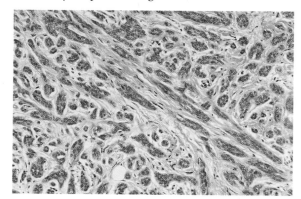

FIG. 5-33. High magnification of Figure 5-32

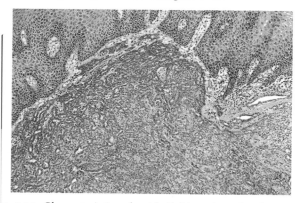

FIG. 5-34. Characteristic subepithelial location of polymorphous low-grade adenocarcinoma

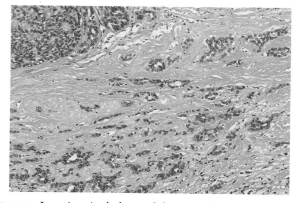

FIG. 5-35. Invasive single-layered ducts, polymorphous low-grade adenocarcinoma

■ Polymorphous Low-Grade Adenocarcinoma

This is, as the name implies, a low-grade malignancy. It has a relatively slow course, with a risk of local recurrence and infrequent metastasis. It appears almost exclusively in minor salivary glands, particularly those in the palate. It occurs during middle and late age and has no gender predilection. It typically presents as a painless swelling, usually without ulceration.

The microscopic interpretation is occasionally difficult because of polymorphous microscopic patterns (Figs. 5–32 through 5–36). It has been confused with adenoid cystic carcinoma, mixed tumor, and monomorphic adenoma. The following features are characteristic of this lesion: nonencapsulation, infiltrative growth, single-layered ducts, cords, and nests. Streaming, cribriform, solid, and syncytial patterns are made by uniform cells with perineural infiltration around small nerve twigs and rare mitotic figures.

Wide excision is generally recommended for treatment of polymorphous low-grade adenocarcinoma. Perineural invasion does not apparently affect prognosis. Prognosis is generally good.

■ Adenoid Cystic Carcinoma

This malignancy of both minor and major salivary glands has a reasonably good short-term prognosis but a particularly poor long-term prognosis. Oral lesions typically appear in the palate as asymptomatic masses that are occasionally ulcerated. Their rate of growth is slow but persistent. They have a propensity for nerve invasion and may cause facial paralysis when occurring in the parotid region. Spread along the perineural/intraneural spaces is believed to be an important factor in recurrence. This lesion occurs in adults and older adults, and there is no gender predilection. Spread to distant organs, such as the lung, seems to be more common than metastasis to regional lymph nodes.

The characteristic cribriform or "Swiss cheese" pattern that characterizes this lesion may be a very prominent or a somewhat obscure feature. This pattern, nonetheless, must be found to make a definitive microscopic diagnosis. Other patterns seen in this neoplasm include a tubular-trabecular pattern and a solid basaloid pattern. Lesions composed predominantly of a solid basaloid pattern are believed to have a poorer overall outcome.

Tumor cells are relatively uniform and show little nuclear atypia. Mitotic figures are rarely seen. Diagnosis is based primarily on pattern recognition (Figs. 5–37 through 5–43). The characteristic microscopic features of adenoid cystic carcinoma are summarized as follows: cribriform, tubular, trabecular, and solid patterns, areas showing distinct and separate (cookie cutter) islands of tumor, retraction spaces around islands, and bilayered ducts often with peripheral clear cells (actin positive).

Wide surgical excision is the treatment of choice. Radical removal may be justified to obtain surgical margins that are free of tumor. Radiation therapy may have a role in tumor control as well. The overall 5-year survival rate is approximately 70%; however, at 15 years, the rate drops to 10%.

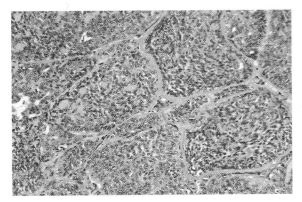

FIG. 5–36. Polymorphous low-grade adenocarcinoma, solid pattern

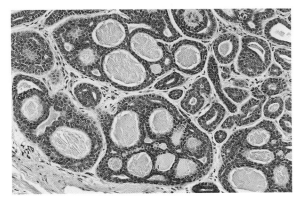

FIG. 5–37. Adenoid cystic carcinoma, cribriform pattern

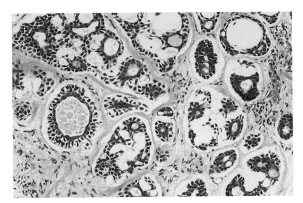

FIG. 5–38. Adenoid cystic carcinoma with clear cells

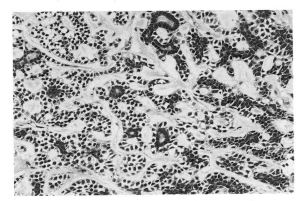

FIG. 5–39. Adenoid cystic carcinoma with clear cells

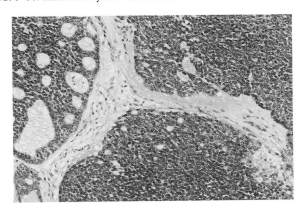

FIG. 5–40. Adenoid cystic carcinoma, solid pattern

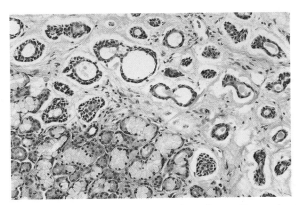

FIG. 5–41. Adenoid cystic carcinoma invading salivary gland

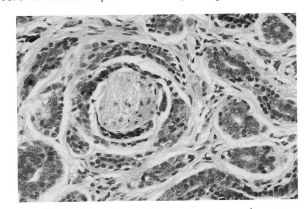

FIG. 5–42. Adenoid cystic carcinoma in perineural space

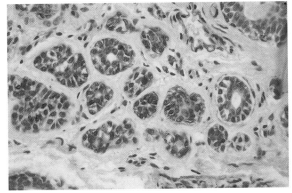

FIG. 5–43. Smooth muscle actin stain of adenoid cystic carcinoma

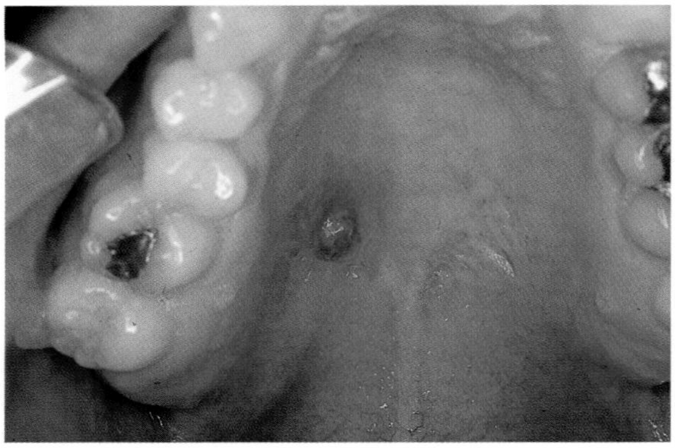

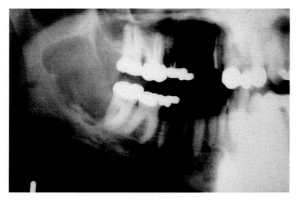

FIG. 5–44. Mucoepidermoid carcinoma of palate

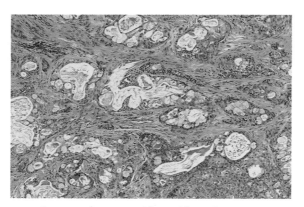

FIG. 5–45. Central mucoepidermoid carcinoma of mandible

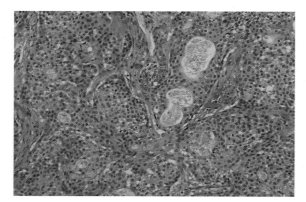

FIG. 5–46. Low-grade mucoepidermoid carcinoma

■ Mucoepidermoid Carcinoma

Malignancies of minor salivary glands occur most commonly in the palate as lumps or ulcerated lumps. Mucoepidermoid carcinoma is the most common malignancy of both minor and major salivary glands. Polymorphous low-grade adenocarcinoma is the second most common and adenoid cystic carcinoma the third most common malignancy of minor glands.

Mucoepidermoid carcinomas are usually seen in adults, although the tumor has been described in children. This neoplasm is most commonly seen in the palate (Fig. 5–44), but it is occasionally found centrally within the jaw, usually the mandible (Fig. 5–45). Mucoepidermoid carcinomas are graded into low, intermediate, and high grades. Low-grade lesions, the most common, are composed of numerous microcystic spaces with abundant mucus-secreting cells (Fig. 5–46). High-grade lesions contain few mucus-producing cells, few cystic spaces, and a more solid lobular pattern. Cellular atypia may also be seen in high-grade lesions. Lesions that are microscopically between low and high grade are considered intermediate-grade mucoepidermoid carcinomas (Fig. 5–47). Clear cell change is occasionally found in mucoepidermoid carcinomas, due to fixation artifact (Fig. 5–48).

The histologic grades of mucoepidermoid carcinomas translate to biologic behavior and prognosis. The overall 5-year survival rate for low-grade lesions is greater than 90%; for high-grade lesions, the survival rate approximates 40%. Surgery is the treatment of choice, with radiation playing a secondary but important role. Local recurrence is more likely than local lymph node metastasis with these lesions.

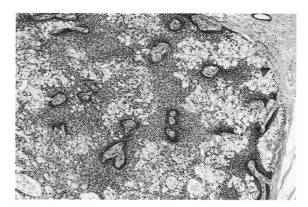

FIG. 5–47. Intermediate-grade mucoepidermoid carcinoma

FIG. 5–48. Mucoepidermoid carcinoma with clear cell change

CHAPTER 5: Salivary Gland Lesions ■ *Adenocarcinomas*

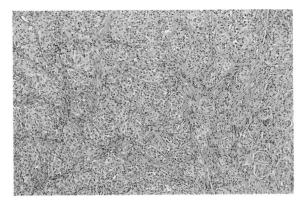

FIG. 5–49. Clear cell carcinoma

■ Clear Cell Carcinoma

Clear cell tumors of salivary gland can be divided into clear cell carcinoma, epimyoepithelial carcinoma, and artifactual change in other tumors (acinic cell carcinoma, oncocytoma, mucoepidermoid carcinoma).

Clear cell carcinoma is a low-grade malignancy predominantly of minor salivary glands. It is characterized by trabeculae, cords, and islands of clear cells that contain glycogen (PAS positive) but not mucin (Figs. 5–49 and 5–50). Supporting stroma is occasionally hyalinized. There is minimal cytologic atypia, and mitotic figures are rare. The lesion is infiltrative. Immunohistochemically, tumor cells express keratin but not S-100 protein or smooth muscle actin, which would be expected in cells with myoepithelial differentiation. Treatment of choice is surgical excision. Both local recurrences and metastasis to local lymph nodes have been described.

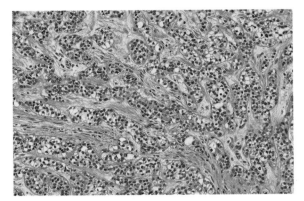

FIG. 5–50. Clear cell carcinoma

■ Epimyoepithelial Carcinoma

This neoplasm appears as a biphasic proliferation of dark cells surrounded by optically clear cells (Fig. 5–51). The pattern is trabecular or nodular, with attempts at duct formation. Epithelial and myoepithelial differentiation have been substantiated by immunohistochemical and ultrastructural studies. This rare malignancy of major and minor salivary glands is generally classified as having intermediate-grade behavior.

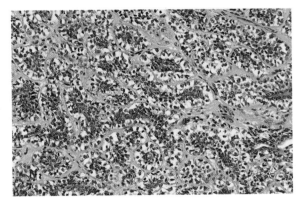

FIG. 5–51. Epimyoepithelial carcinoma

■ Acinic Cell Carcinoma

Acinic cell carcinoma is rarely seen arising from minor salivary glands. The tumor cells mimic acinar cells by their production of PAS-positive zymogen granules (Fig. 5–52). Solid, trabecular, papillary cystic, and follicular patterns have been described. Zones of clear cell change, due presumably to fixation artifact, may be seen (Fig. 5–53).

This is a slow-growing, low-grade malignancy. Prognosis is generally very good, although recurrences often occur by 5, and sometimes 15, years after treatment. Local recurrence is the rule, although metastasis to local nodes and distant organs can be seen.

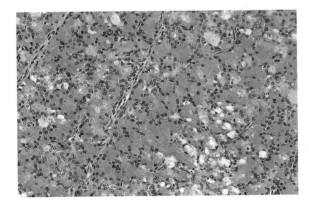

FIG. 5–52. Acinic cell carcinoma

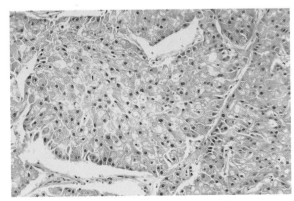

FIG. 5–53. Acinic cell carcinoma with clear cell change

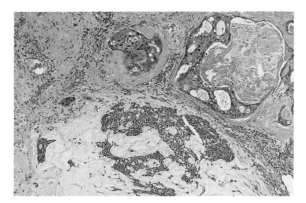

FIG. 5–54. Carcinoma ex mixed tumor

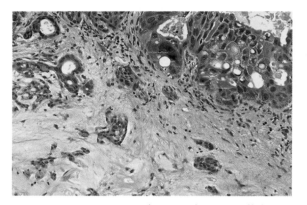

FIG. 5–55. Carcinoma ex mixed tumor showing cellular atypia

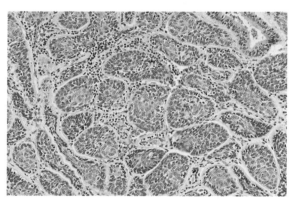

FIG. 5–56. Basal cell adenocarcinoma

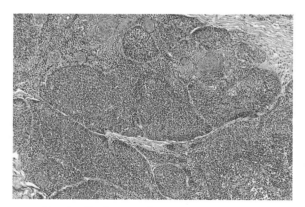

FIG. 5–57. Basal cell adenocarcinoma

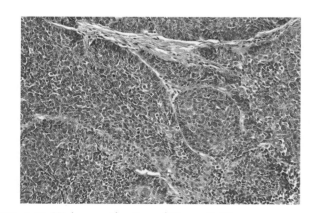

FIG. 5–58. High magnification of Figure 5–57

■ Carcinoma Ex Mixed Tumor

This represents an epithelial malignancy arising in a pre-existing mixed tumor. The malignant component shows cellular atypia and is invasive (Figs. 5–54 and 5–55). Metastatic deposits resemble squamous cell carcinoma. This type of malignancy typically occurs after a decade or more of persistent mixed tumor, or after multiple surgeries to eliminate a benign mixed tumor. This is predominantly a major salivary gland malignancy, although many have been described in minor salivary glands. It is regarded as a high-grade neoplasm.

In rare instances, both epithelial and mesenchymal components of a mixed tumor may become malignant. These neoplasms are referred to as malignant mixed tumors. These are also high-grade neoplasms.

■ Basal Cell Adenocarcinoma

This is a rare tumor, predominantly of major salivary glands. It is regarded as the malignant counterpart of basal cell adenoma. It is composed of basaloid cells that exhibit an infiltrative growth pattern. Nests, cords, and solid zones of basal cells are seen (Fig. 5–56 through 5–58). Often there is a biphasic appearance of small compact cells lying peripheral to larger polygonal cells. Local recurrence may be seen, as well as metastasis. This is usually a low-grade malignancy.

Cysts and Cystlike Lesions

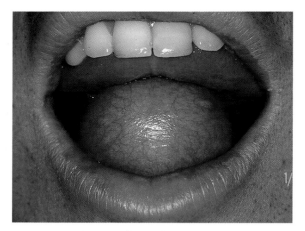

FIG. 6–1. Dermoid cyst in floor of mouth

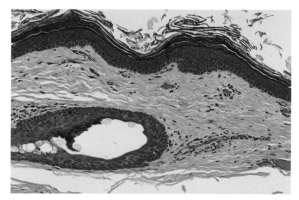

FIG. 6–2. Dermoid cyst with hair in wall

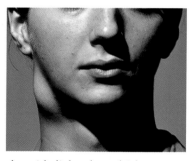

FIG. 6–3. Lymphoepithelial or branchial cyst

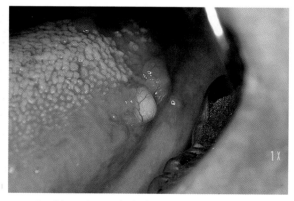

FIG. 6–4. Oral lymphoepithelial cyst of lateral tongue

■ Dermoid Cyst

This is a soft tissue developmental cyst that occurs occasionally in the ovary and infrequently in the midline of the neck or anterior floor of the mouth. The lining is derived from multipotential cells with the capability of giving rise to tissues of one or more germ layers. If the cyst wall contains cutaneous structures, it is called *dermoid cyst*. If tissues such as cartilage, muscle, and brain from other germ layers are present, it is called *teratoma*.

Clinically, when dermoid cysts develop superior to the mylohyoid muscle, the tongue is displaced, leaving a mass in the oral floor (Fig. 6–1). When developing inferior to the mylohyoid and geniohyoid muscles, mass appears in the midline of the neck. Treatment is surgical excision.

Microscopically, these cysts are lined by keratinized stratified squamous epithelium. The diagnostic feature is the presence of secondary skin structures; hair and sebaceous glands (Fig. 6–2). The accumulation of sebum and keratin in the cyst lumen gives the lesion a doughy consistency when palpated.

■ Lymphoepithelial Cyst

This developmental cyst may occur in the lateral neck or intraorally in lymphoid deposits. When in the neck, the terms *branchial (cleft) cyst* and *cervical lymphoepithelial cyst* are used. The origin of the epithelium lining this cyst is believed to be either embryonic epithelial remnants of the branchial clefts or epithelial rests trapped in developing lymphoid tissue.

This neck cyst typically occurs in teenagers and young adults as a slow-growing asymptomatic mass in the lateral neck, anterior to the sternocleidomastoid muscle (Fig. 6–3). Oral lymphoepithelial cysts are seen at any age in the lateral tongue, floor of mouth, or tonsilar pillars (Fig. 6–4). They are less than 1 cm in diameter and appear yellow. These lesions appear similar to ectopic lymphoid tissue and represent, in some cases, lymphoid hyperplasia associated with plugging of lymphoid crypts.

Microscopically, these cysts are lined by stratified squamous or pseudostratified ciliated epithelium. The diagnostic feature is the presence of normal lymphoid tissue in the supporting connective tissue wall (Fig. 6–5).

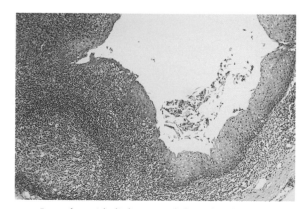

FIG. 6–5. Lymphoepithelial cyst with lymphoid tissue in wall

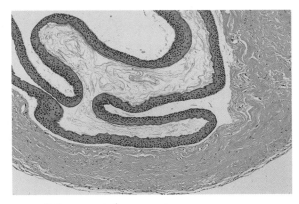

FIG. 6–28. Odontogenic keratocyst

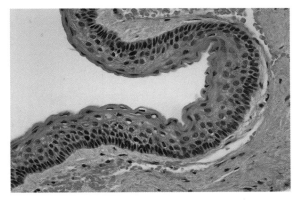

FIG. 6–29. Odontogenic keratocyst

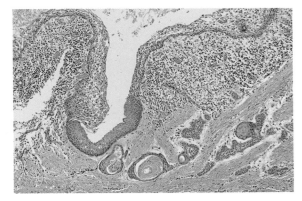

FIG. 6–30. Odontogenic keratocyst

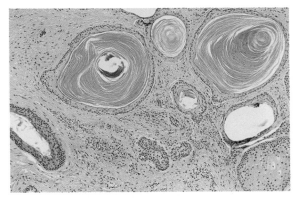

FIG. 6–31. Odontogenic keratocyst with "daughter" cysts

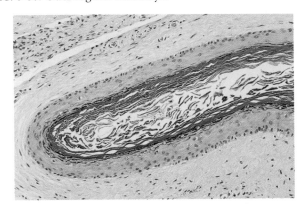

FIG. 6–32. Orthokeratinized odontogenic cyst

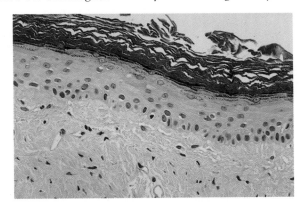

FIG. 6–33. Orthokeratinized odontogenic cyst

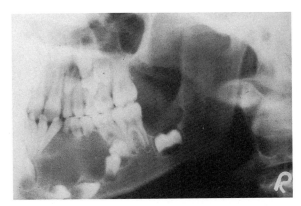

FIG. 6–34. Keratocysts in nevoid–basal cell carcinoma syndrome

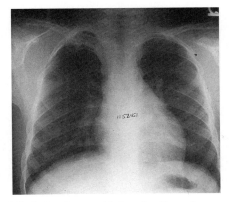

FIG. 6–35. Rib fusion in nevoid–basal cell carcinoma syndrome

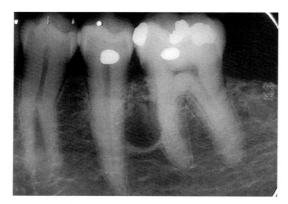

FIG. 6–36. Lateral root cyst

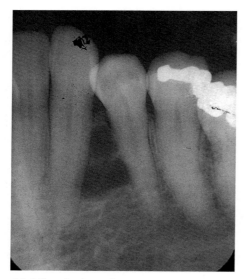

FIG. 6–37. Multilocular lateral root cyst

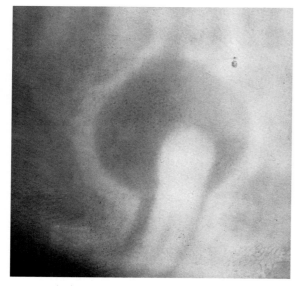

FIG. 6–38. Calcifying odontogenic cyst

■ Lateral Periodontal Cyst

This is a developmental cyst that occurs along the lateral root surface of a vital tooth, especially in the premolar region (Figs. 6–36 and 6–37). This lesion generally remains small, but it may present as a loculated lucency. The lining is distinctive, consisting of nonkeratinized thin (two or three cell layers) epithelium with focal thickenings (Figs. 6–39 and 6–40). Inflammatory cells are scant. Loculated versions are sometimes called *botryoid odontogenic cysts*. There is also a gingival soft tissue counterpart to the lateral periodontal cyst known simply as *gingival cyst*.

■ Calcifying Odontogenic Cyst

This is a developmental lesion that, because of occasional aggressive behavior and occasional solid gross and microscopic patterns, has been viewed by some as a neoplasm, prompting the term "odontogenic ghost cell tumor." It shows a predilection for females and the maxilla. It occasionally is seen in the gingiva. It may be unilocular or multilocular, and may show areas of opacification due to partial calcification of keratinized lining cells (Fig. 6–38). The distinctive microscopic feature of this lesion, be it cystic or solid, is "ghost cell" keratinization of the epithelial lining (Figs. 6–41 and 6–42). The keratin may undergo dystrophic calcification and may incite a foreign body reaction in the cyst wall, giving it features similar to the pilomatrixoma of the skin.

■ Glandular Odontogenic Cyst

This is a rare and recently described developmental jaw lesion that mimics superficially a mucus-producing salivary gland tumor microscopically. It is seen in adults in any jaw site, although anterior regions are favored. This multilocular cyst is lined by nonkeratinized epithelium with focal thickenings composed of mucus and clear cells in a pseudoglandular pattern (Figs. 6–43 and 6–44). This lesion has shown local aggressiveness and has recurrence potential.

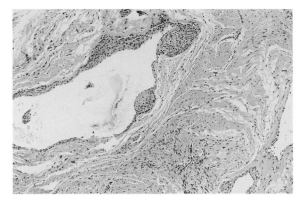

FIG. 6–39. Lateral root cyst

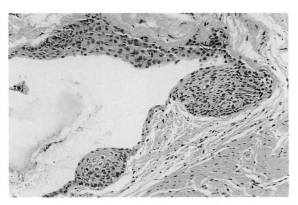

FIG. 6–40. High magnification of Figure 6–39 showing epithelial tufts

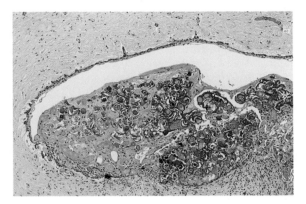

FIG. 6–41. Calcifying odontogenic cyst

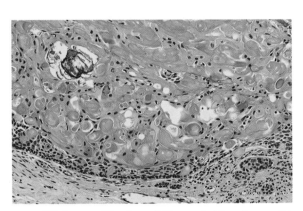

FIG. 6–42. High magnification of Figure 6–41—ghost cell keratinization

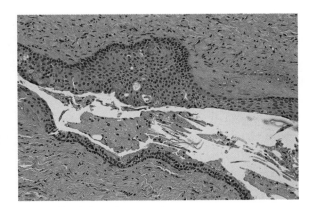

FIG. 6–43. Glandular odontogenic cyst

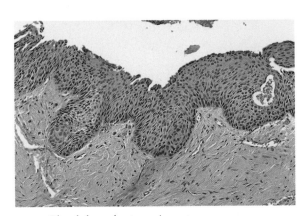

FIG. 6–44. Glandular odontogenic cyst

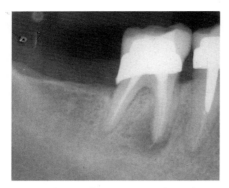

FIG. 6–45. Periapical granuloma (nonvital tooth)

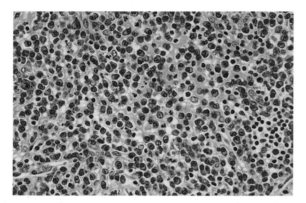

FIG. 6–46. Inflammatory response in a periapical granuloma

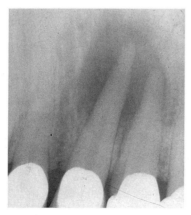

FIG. 6–47. Periapical cyst (nonvital tooth)

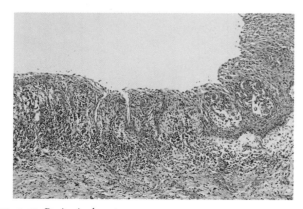

FIG. 6–48. Periapical cyst

■ Periapical Granuloma

Periapical granulomas and cysts have a common etiology. They are associated with nonvital teeth whose necrotic pulps stimulate an inflammatory response in the periodontal ligament and bone at the tooth apex (Fig. 6–45). Once the inflammatory stimulus is removed (tooth extraction or endodontic filling), the repair process continues, ultimately leading to regeneration of bone in the area.

A periapical or dental granuloma represents a focus of granulation tissue and inflammatory cells that have replaced apical bone (Fig. 6–46). Occasionally, a marked plasma cell infiltrate is seen, mimicking or suggesting multiple myeloma. Periapical granuloma is to be distinguished from granulomatous inflammation in which there is an abundance of macrophages, as in tuberculosis or sarcoidosis. A periapical granuloma may develop from low-grade, sustained chronic inflammation or from a quiescent abscess that has not been treated. Variable amounts of scar are seen in periapical granulomas and represent advanced repair. Occasionally, when cortical perforation is present, osteogenesis does not occur and the lesion remains as a *periapical scar*, even in the presence of an adequate root canal filling. Also, if there is open communication between the tooth apex and oral cavity (e.g., through a carious lesion), the microaerophilic bacterium Actinomyces, found in the oral flora, can colonize the inflamed periapical tissues. This variation of periapical granuloma can result in actinomycosis of the jaw.

■ Periapical Cyst

A periapical cyst is a pathologic space lined by epithelium at the apex of a nonvital tooth (Fig. 6–47). The epithelium proliferates in a pre-existing periapical granuloma due to inflammatory stimulation of the ubiquitous rests of Malassez found in the apical periodontal ligament. Microscopic examination shows a variable picture ranging from partial to complete epithelization of the periapex (Fig. 6–48). Diagnosis is dependent upon when, in this process, the lesion is biopsied and on how the pathologist defines periapical cyst. The subjectivity associated with microscopic diagnosis in all likelihood accounts for the wide range of periapical cyst incidence (10% to 50%) in the literature.

It is generally agreed that once a periapical granuloma becomes well epithelialized, complete bony healing is unlikely after root canal therapy alone. Whether a partially epithelized periapical granuloma can heal after a canal is filled is still unknown, although it is likely that some can. Probably most of the endodontically treated teeth in which periapical lesions persist (approximately 10% to 20% of cases) are related to cystic change of a periapical granuloma. Also, some persistent lesions may be associated with incompletely filled canals and/or apical foreign material. Although large lesions are more likely to be cysts, it is not possible radiographically to distinguish a periapical granuloma from a periapical cyst.

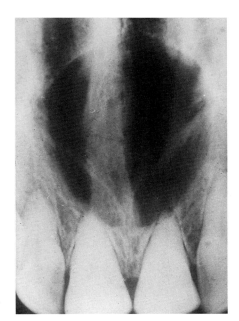

FIG. 6–49. Nasopalatine canal cyst

■ Nasopalatine Canal Cyst

Also known as incisive canal cyst, this is a relatively common lesion that is derived from proliferation of the epithelial remnants of the vestigial nasopalatine ducts (Figs. 6–49 through 6–51). It is probably the only "true" non-odontogenic cyst that occurs in the jaws: the globulomaxillary cyst and the midmandibular cyst have been deleted from classifications because their proposed embryologic origin is unsubstantiated. Lesions in these sites have been shown to be other known odontogenic cysts and tumors. Also, the so-called midpalatine cyst is believed to represent a large nasopalatine cyst.

The nasopalatine cyst is always radiolucent and found in the midline of the maxilla in association with vital teeth. When the diameter of the radiographic image of the nasopalatine canal exceeds 7 mm, cystic change should be strongly suspected. The epithelial lining ranges from stratified squamous to pseudostratified ciliated. The neurovascular contents of the nasopalatine canal are usually seen in the cyst wall.

■ Static Bone Cyst

Also known as *Stafne bone cyst*, this represents an anatomic defect of the mandible, which has a cystlike appearance radiographically (Fig. 6–52). The defect is an invagination of the lingual surface of the mandible. The space created is filled with the contents of the floor of the mouth, usually salivary gland or adipose tissue. The characteristic location is the molar area, subjacent to the mandibular canal. The radiographic image is usually diagnostic, and the lesion requires no biopsy or treatment.

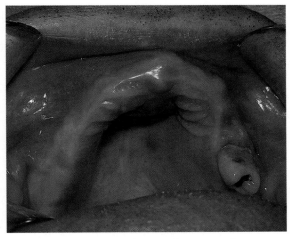

FIG. 6–50. Oral expression of nasopalatine canal cyst

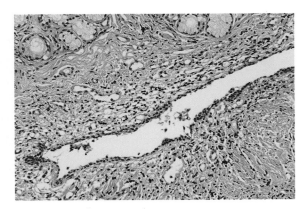

FIG. 6–51. Nasopalatine canal cyst

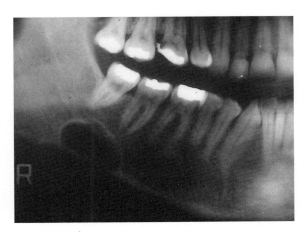

FIG. 6–52. Static bone cyst

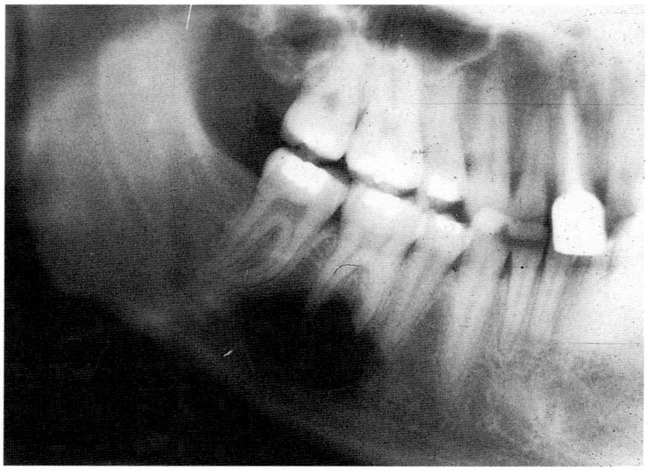

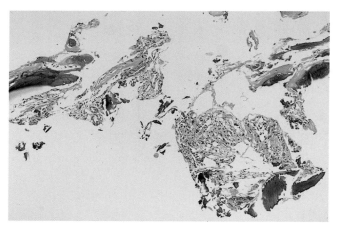

FIG. 6-53. Traumatic bone cyst

■ Traumatic Bone Cyst

Also known as simple bone cyst, this is a pseudocyst (no epithelial lining) that represents a bony dead space. Although trauma is suspected as an etiologic factor, this has not been proven. The lesion is believed to develop from abnormal healing of intrabony hemorrhage. The natural history has not been elucidated, but it is suspected that these lesions are capable of resolution without surgical intervention. Nonetheless, exploration is usually done to rule out other more important lesions. Traumatic bone cysts are typically seen as unilocular lucencies in the mandibles of teenagers (Fig. 6-53). Surgical specimens are in the form of bits of fibrous tissue and bone from the wall of the dead space (Fig. 6-54). It is prudent to have clinicopathologic correlation. Once the lesion is diagnosed, no treatment is required because the dead space fills with blood, which undergoes organization and ossification.

■ Hematopoietic Bone Marrow Defect

This condition presents as an ill-defined and often loculated lucency and represents a focus of hematopoiesis in an atypical site. Most appear in the posterior mandible, particularly in an edentulous space after the extraction of a tooth (Figs. 6-55 and 6-56). The pathogenesis is unknown but may be related to abnormal healing or simply ectopic marrow. Although lesions are biopsied for diagnostic purposes, no treatment is necessary.

FIG. 6-54. Tissue fragments from traumatic bone cyst wall

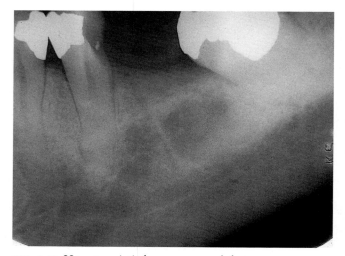

FIG. 6-55. Hematopoietic bone marrow defect

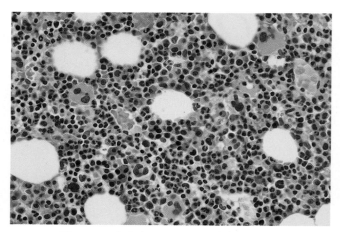

FIG. 6-56. Hematopoietic bone marrow defect

CHAPTER 7

Odontogenic Tumors

Epithelial

Ameloblastoma

Cystic Ameloblastomas

Malignant Ameloblastomas

Calcifying Epithelial Odontogenic Tumor

Squamous Odontogenic Tumor

Clear Cell Odontogenic Tumor (Carcinoma)

Adenomatoid Odontogenic Tumor

Mesenchymal

Odontogenic Myxoma

Central Odontogenic Fibroma

Cementoblastoma

Periapical Cemento-Osseous Dysplasia

Florid Osseous Dysplasia

Mixed Epithelial-Mesenchymal

Ameloblastic Fibroma

Odontoma

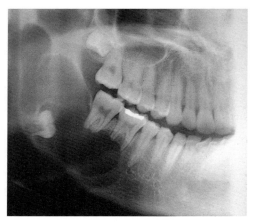

FIG. 7–1. Ameloblastoma associated with impacted third molar

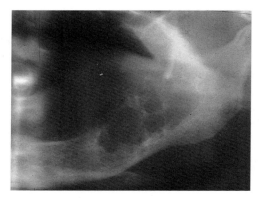

FIG. 7–2. Multilocular ameloblastoma in edentulous mandible

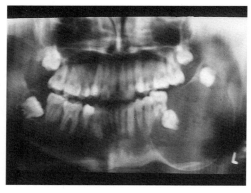

FIG. 7–3. Expansive ameloblastoma of posterior mandible

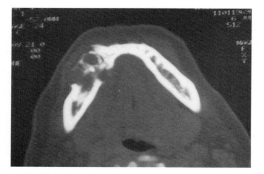

FIG. 7–4. CT scan of loculated mandibular ameloblastoma

■ Ameloblastoma

This is a benign but often aggressive neoplasm of odontogenic origin. Microscopically, it mimics the ameloblasts and stellate reticulum that ordinarily give rise to enamel. No hard tissue is formed by the tumor cells.

PATHOGENESIS

Ameloblastomas arise from either neoplastic transformation of odontogenic cyst epithelium or from residual epithelial rests left over from the formation of teeth, such as remnants of the enamel organ (reduced enamel epithelium) found over the crown of an unerupted tooth, remnants of Hertwig's epithelial root sheath (rests of Malassez) in the periodontal ligament, or remnants of the dental lamina (rests of Serres). Ameloblastomas may be confused clinically with other jaw lesions and occasionally with infiltrating neoplasms of the maxillary sinus, particularly those of salivary gland origin.

CLINICAL FEATURES

Ameloblastomas typically occur around the age of 40 years; children are rarely affected. Odontogenic tumors that are more likely to appear in children are adenomatoid odontogenic tumor and ameloblastic fibroma (both of which have decidedly different microscopic features and biologic behaviors). Ameloblastoma may appear anywhere in the jaws, although the molar-ramus area of the mandible is the favored location (Figs. 7–1 through 7–4). Affected patients are asymptomatic, and lesions are usually discovered during routine radiographic examination or because of jaw swelling. Radiographically, ameloblastomas usually appear as well-defined unilocular or multilocular lucencies. They characteristically exhibit slow but unrelenting and destructive growth.

MICROSCOPIC FEATURES

Ameloblastomas mimic enamel organ (Fig. 7–5). They also exhibit a remarkable histologic similarity to basal cell carcinoma. These shared features are likely related to shared histogenetic origins. Numerous histologic patterns (no biologic differences) may be seen in ameloblastomas (Figs. 7–6 through 7–10). The common denominator to all ameloblastomas is well-differentiated palisaded cells found around the periphery of nests, strands, and networks of epithelium. Nuclei of the palisaded cells are typically polarized away from the basement membrane. Budding of epithelium from these proliferative nests and strands is also characteristic of this lesion. Palisading cells and budding epithelium are found in all microscopic subtypes (follicular, cystic, plexiform, desmoplastic, acanthomatous, granular cell). Keratinization in the form of ghost cells may be seen in ameloblastomas as well as other odontogenic tumors and cysts (particularly the calcifying odontogenic cyst).

Extraosseous gingival tumors (*peripheral ameloblastoma*) are very infrequently seen (Figs. 7–11 and 7–12). These lesions have microscopic features similar to their intrabony counterparts. However, they do not exhibit the clinical aggressiveness associated with central lesions.

Ameloblastomas require at least surgical excision, if not resection. Recurrence rates of 50% to 90% have been associated with lesions treated by curettage alone.

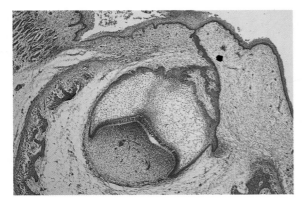

FIG. 7–5. Mandibular enamel organ in 22-week fetus

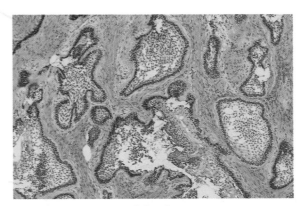

FIG. 7–6. Ameloblastoma—follicular pattern

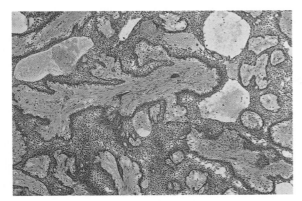

FIG. 7–7. Ameloblastoma—plexiform or reticular pattern

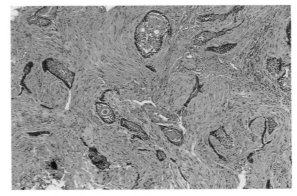

FIG. 7–8. Desmoplastic ameloblastoma

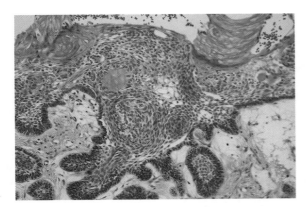

FIG. 7–9. Ameloblastoma with ghost cell keratinization

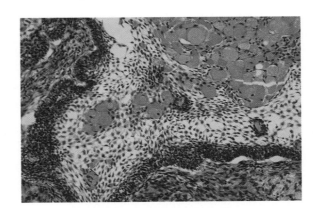

FIG. 7–10. Ameloblastoma with granular cells

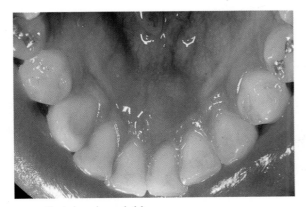

FIG. 7–11. Peripheral ameloblastoma

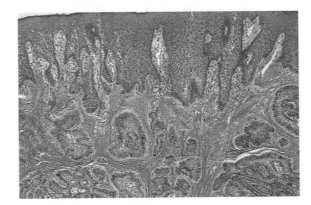

FIG. 7–12. Peripheral ameloblastoma

CHAPTER 7: Odontogenic Tumors ■ *Epithelial*

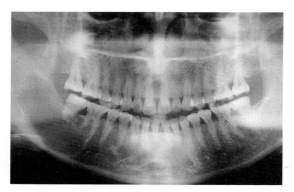

FIG. 7–13. Cystic ameloblastoma of mandible

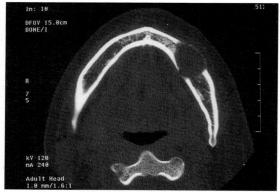

FIG. 7–14. CT scan of mandibular cystic ameloblastoma

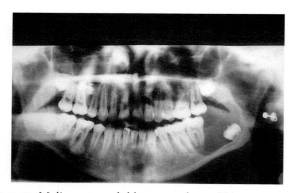

FIG. 7–15. Malignant ameloblastoma of mandible

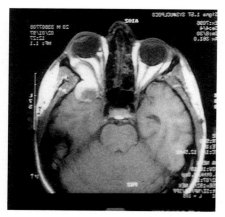

FIG. 7–16. CT scan of malignant ameloblastoma

Cystic Ameloblastoma

This biologic subtype of ameloblastoma is also known as unicystic ameloblastoma and occasionally as plexiform unicystic ameloblastoma. It has been separated from the solid type because it appears at a younger age, has a lower recurrence rate, and requires less aggressive surgery to cure. Diagnosis is often difficult, frequently being made retrospectively.

CLINICAL FEATURES
Cystic ameloblastomas usually occur in the second to third decades and in the mandibular molar area. They are entirely cystic and consist usually of a single space, although some may be loculated. Radiographically, these lesions are lucent, with well-defined margins. They may appear at the apex of a tooth or around the crown of an impacted tooth. They are usually small, although they can reach several centimeters in size (Fig. 7–13). Cystic ameloblastomas can occasionally expand or perforate jaw cortex. Figure 7–14 is a CT scan of such a lesion.

MICROSCOPIC FEATURES
This is a deceptively innocent-appearing lesion that is often underdiagnosed as simple odontogenic cyst. The diagnosis is often made in retrospect when the lesion recurs. Figures 7–17 through 7–20 represent recurrent cystic ameloblastomas. Features that help in microscopic diagnosis include basal cell palisading, epithelial invagination, epithelial edema, and cell dysadhesion. Clinicopathologic correlation is very helpful and often essential.

Malignant Ameloblastomas

The malignant ameloblastomas have been divided into two subtypes: *ameloblastic carcinoma*, in which primary and metastatic lesions show dedifferentiation with cytologic atypia; and *malignant ameloblastoma*, in which the metastatic lesion microscopically resembles ameloblastoma. There is also another malignancy of odontogenic origin, called *primary intraosseous carcinoma*, that may rarely occur centrally in the jaws. This lesion, thought to arise from odontogenic rests in bone, looks like squamous cell carcinoma and shows no microscopic features of ameloblastoma.

CLINICAL FEATURES
Malignant ameloblastoma (Figs. 7–15 and 7–16) and ameloblastic carcinoma occur at a younger age than ameloblastoma and are usually seen in the mandible. Metastasis is typically to the lung and occasionally to local lymph nodes.

MICROSCOPIC FEATURES
The three sequential photomicrographs (Figs. 7–21 to 7–23) taken over a 6-year period show the dedifferentiation of the ameloblastic carcinoma illustrated in panoramic film and CT scan. Note how the last specimen (Fig. 7–23) bears little resemblance to the original tumor (Fig. 7–21). Figure 7–24 shows a malignant ameloblastoma metastatic to the lung. The tumor shows the histologic pattern of ameloblastoma.

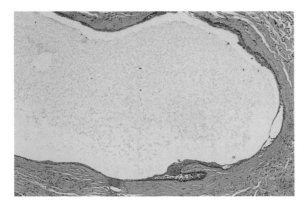

FIG. 7–17. Recurrent cystic ameloblastoma

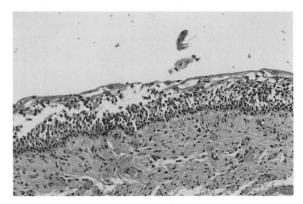

FIG. 7–18. Recurrent cystic ameloblastoma

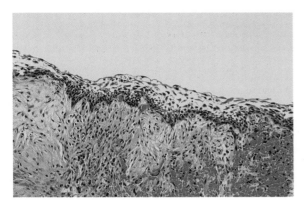

FIG. 7–19. Recurrent cystic ameloblastoma

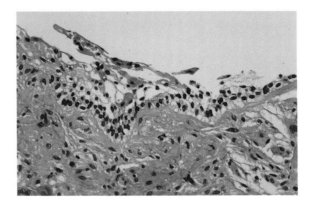

FIG. 7–20. Recurrent cystic ameloblastoma

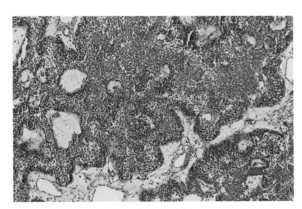

FIG. 7–21. Original biopsy of ameloblastic carcinoma

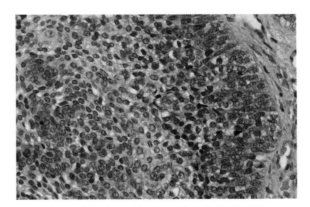

FIG. 7–22. Ameloblastic carcinoma after 6 years

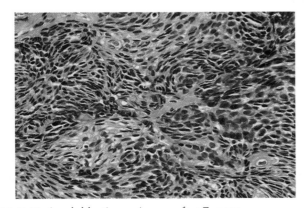

FIG. 7–23. Ameloblastic carcinoma after 7 years

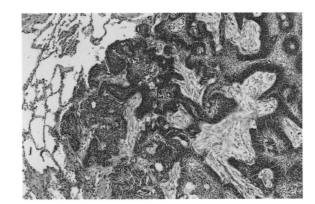

FIG. 7–24. Malignant ameloblastoma in lung

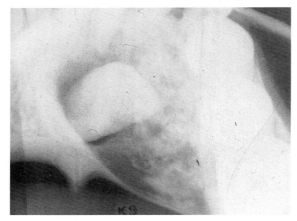
FIG. 7–25. Calcifying odontogenic tumor surrounding impacted tooth

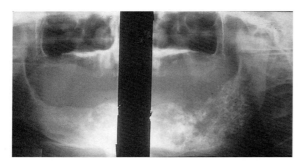
FIG. 7–26. CEOT in posterior edentulous mandible

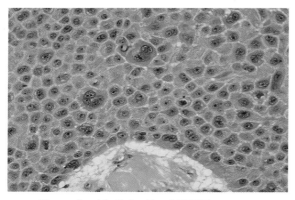
FIG. 7–27. Unusual epithelial cells of CEOT

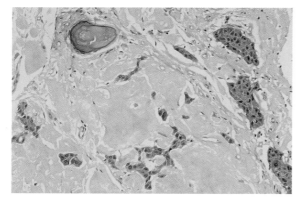
FIG. 7–28. CEOT with high amyloid content

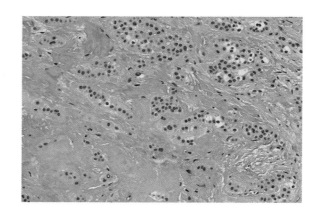

■ Calcifying Epithelial Odontogenic Tumor

Calcifying epithelial odontogenic tumor (CEOT), also known as *Pindborg tumor*, is a rare odontogenic tumor of disputed pathogenesis.

CLINICAL AND RADIOGRAPHIC FEATURES
This tumor occurs in the same age range (30 to 50 years) and in the same jaw sites (posterior mandible favored) as ameloblastoma. It is a slow-growing, benign neoplasm. It may be unilocular or multilocular (Figs. 7–25 and 7–26). Because of focal areas of calcification, the radiographic picture is occasionally a mixed pattern. Rarely, this tumor occurs in the soft tissues of the gingiva (peripheral CEOT).

MICROSCOPIC FEATURES
CEOT consists of sheets of large epithelioid cells with zones of amyloid deposits, which may show dystrophic calcification (Figs. 7–27 to 7–29). The tumor cells may exhibit considerable range in nuclear size and shape, but mitotic figures are not seen. The ratio of epithelium to extracellular product can be quite variable from one tumor to another. Occasionally, the epithelial cells exhibit clear cytoplasm.

TREATMENT
Behavior is generally thought to be less aggressive than ameloblastoma. Therefore, a less aggressive surgical approach is used to treat these lesions. A small percentage may recur; re-excision is usually curative.

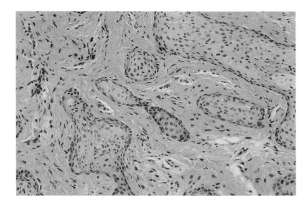

FIG. 7–30. Squamous odontogenic tumor

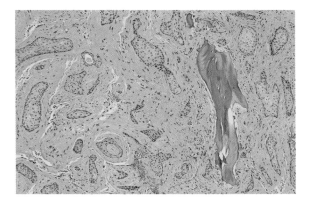

FIG. 7–31. Squamous odontogenic tumor

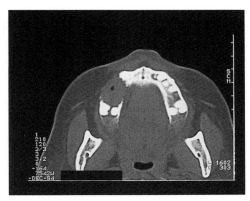

FIG. 7–32. CT scan of clear cell odontogenic tumor of maxilla

■ Squamous Odontogenic Tumor

Squamous odontogenic tumor is a benign odontogenic lesion that, because of its presentation in the alveolar process, is believed to originate from rests of Malassez. It occurs in the mandible and maxilla with equal frequency and may be multiple. In the alveolar process, it is well circumscribed and is usually associated with the roots of teeth. It is typically small and typically appears radiographically as a wedge-shaped lucency at the crest of the alveolar process.

Microscopically, it resembles ameloblastoma (acanthomatous type). It appears as islands of bland squamous epithelium without an inflammatory infiltrate (Fig. 7–30). Peripheral palisades are not seen. The epithelial islands occasionally surround specules of bone (Fig. 7–31). Because it seems to have limited growth potential, conservative surgical treatment is indicated.

■ Clear Cell Odontogenic Tumor (Carcinoma)

This is a rare jaw tumor that some consider to be a carcinoma because of its behavior. Clear cell odontogenic tumor (carcinoma) has been described mostly in women over the age of 60 years. It may cause some pain. Radiographically, the lesion is lucent and either unilocular or multilocular (Fig. 7–32).

Microscopically, nests and cords of clear cells are seen (Figs. 7–33 and 7–34). Some peripheral palisading may be present. Differential diagnosis would include calcifying epithelial odontogenic tumor, central mucoepidermoid carcinoma, metastatic acinic cell carcinoma, metastatic renal cell carcinoma, and ameloblastoma.

This rare lesion has an aggressive biologic behavior. Metastases to lung and regional lymph nodes have been reported.

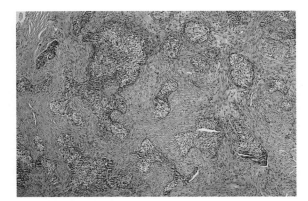

FIG. 7–33. Clear cell odontogenic tumor

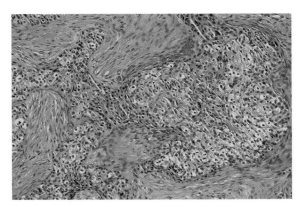

FIG. 7–34. High magnification of Figure 7–33

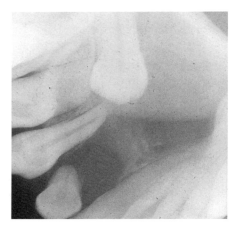

FIG. 7-35. AOT associated with impacted canine

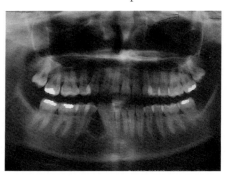

FIG. 7-36. AOT causing divergence of roots of mandibular teeth

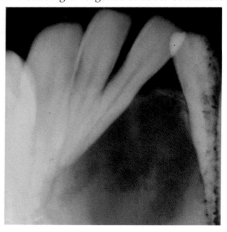

FIG. 7-37. AOT between mandibular incisors

■ Adenomatoid Odontogenic Tumor

The adenomatoid odontogenic tumor (AOT) exhibits pseudoduct formation microscopically. It should not be confused with the distinctively different ameloblastoma.

CLINICAL AND RADIOGRAPHIC FEATURES

AOT is characteristically seen in children and teenagers in the anterior jaws, often in association with impacted teeth (Fig. 7–35). Females are more commonly affected than males. Rarely is it seen over the age of 30 years. This lesion has been seen rarely in the gingiva. Radiographically, AOT is well circumscribed and unilocular. Occasionally, divergence of roots adjacent to the lesion can be seen (Figs. 7–36 and 7–37). Most lesions are radiolucent, but some have opaque islands scattered throughout.

MICROSCOPIC FEATURES

AOT is a well-circumscribed odontogenic epithelial proliferation that shows pseudoduct or rosette formation (Figs. 7–38 through 7–45). The epithelial pattern is lobular and occasionally plexiform. Foci of calcified material, called enameloid, may be seen in the lesion.

TREATMENT

Conservative surgical treatment (curettage) is the treatment for this lesion. It is completely benign and almost never recurs.

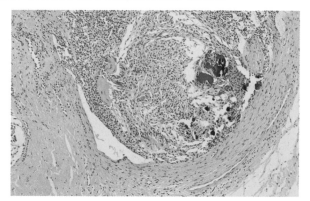

FIG. 7-38. Low magnification of AOT showing capsule

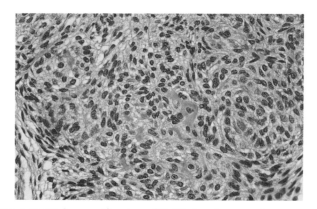

FIG. 7-39. High magnification of 7-38 showing pseudorosettes

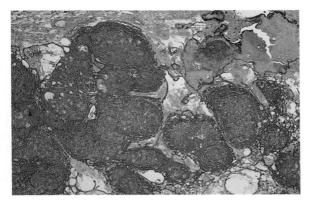

FIG. 7–40. Lobular pattern of AOT

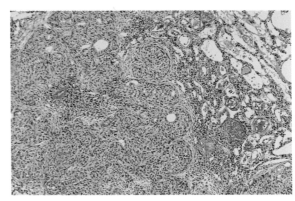

FIG. 7–41. Lobular pattern of AOT

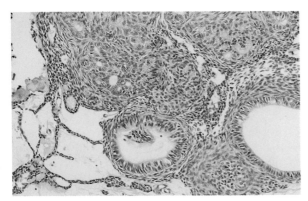

FIG. 7–42. Pseudoducts in AOT

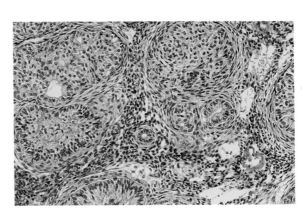

FIG. 7–43. Pseudoducts in AOT

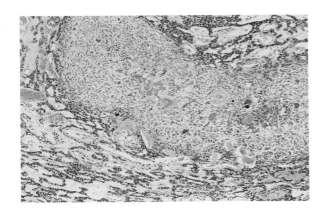

FIG. 7–44. Lobular-plexiform pattern of AOT

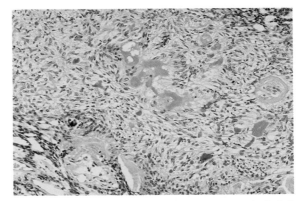

FIG. 7–45. High magnification of 7–44 showing calcified deposits

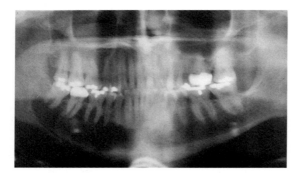

FIG. 7–46. Odontogenic myxoma of mandibular right body

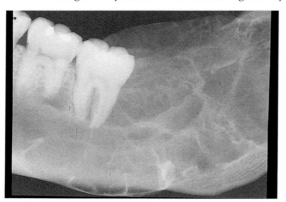

FIG. 7–47. Multilocularity of odontogenic myxoma

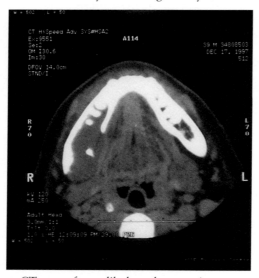

FIG. 7–48. CT scan of mandibular odontogenic myxoma

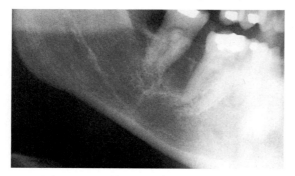

FIG. 7–49. Odontogenic fibroma of mandible

■ Odontogenic Myxoma

This benign and sometimes clinically aggressive tumor mimics microscopically the dental pulp. It occurs typically in adults (mean age 30, range 10 to 50) as a radiolucent lesion, often with small loculations (honeycomb pattern) (Figs. 7–46 to 7–48).

Odontogenic myxoma has a bland myxoid microscopic appearance (Figs. 7–51 and 7–52). If collagen is prominent, the designation of *myxofibroma* may be used (Fig. 7–53). Bony islands, representing residual trabeculae, are found throughout the lesion. Odontogenic epithelial rests are very uncommon in these lesions. If odontogenic rests are found in a myxomatous jaw lesion, follicular sac (normal tissue found around the crowns of unerupted teeth) should be seriously considered. Occasionally, as part of a jaw biopsy, normal dental pulp of a developing tooth may be submitted for microscopic diagnosis. This tissue has the appearance of an odontogenic myxoma except for peripheral columnar-shaped odontoblasts. An accurate clinical history and radiographs can be invaluable in separating follicular sac and normal dental pulp from odontogenic myxoma.

■ Central Odontogenic Fibroma

This is a tumor of adults and appears as a well-defined radiolucency in either jaw (Figs. 7–49 and 7–50). It is not, however, particularly aggressive, and it infrequently recurs after simple curettage.

Microscopically, these lesions are more collagenous than myxomas, and may range from myxofibrous to densely fibrous. Characteristically seen in central odontogenic fibromas are few to many islands and strands of bland odontogenic epithelium (Figs. 7–54 and 7–55). Calcific deposits may also be found. A variant (*granular cell odontogenic fibroma*), in which granular cells are seen in the connective tissue, has been described (Fig. 7–56). The behavior of this tumor does not appear to differ from central odontogenic fibroma. Hyperplastic follicular sacs can occasionally mimic myxomas (Fig. 7–57), and rest proliferation in follicular sacs can occasionally simulate the appearance of odontogenic fibroma (Fig. 7–58).

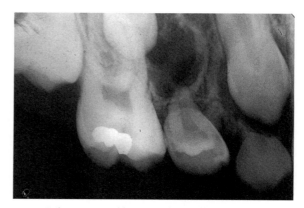

FIG. 7–50. Odontogenic fibroma of maxilla

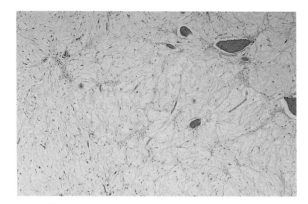

FIG. 7–51. Odontogenic myxoma

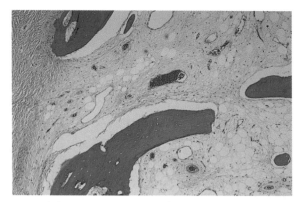

FIG. 7–52. Odontogenic myxoma showing cortical penetration (left)

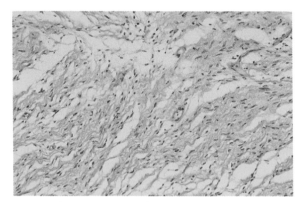

FIG. 7–53. Odontogenic myxofibroma

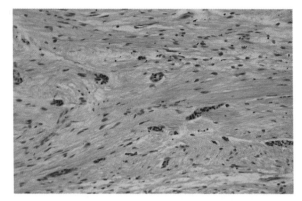

FIG. 7–54. Odontogenic fibroma (note epithelial strands)

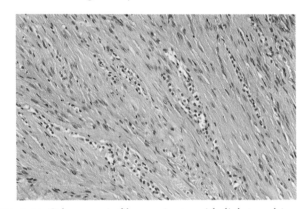

FIG. 7–55. Odontogenic fibroma (note epithelial strands)

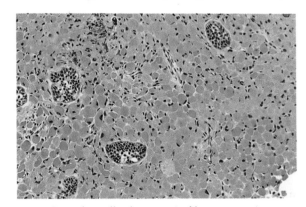

FIG. 7–56. Granular cell odontogenic fibroma

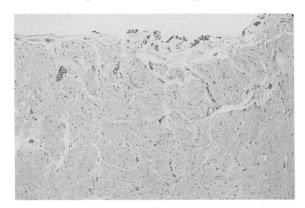

FIG. 7–57. Follicular sac with reduced enamel epithelium (top)

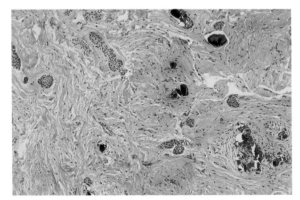

FIG. 7–58. Follicular sac with rests and calcifications

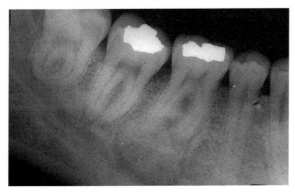

FIG. 7–59. Cementoblastoma

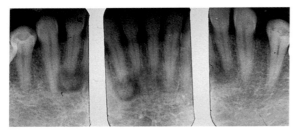

FIG. 7–60. Periapical cemento-osseous dysplasia

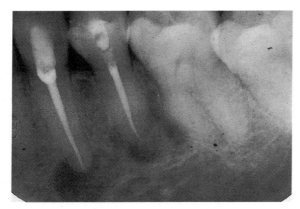

FIG. 7–61. Periapical cemento-osseous dysplasia

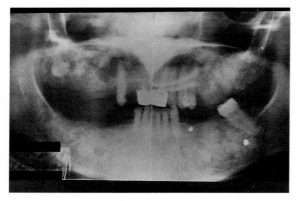

FIG. 7–62. Florid osseous dysplasia

■ Cementoblastoma

Cementoblastoma is a lesion seen in young adults that results in replacement of tooth root with abundant amounts of tumor cementum (Fig. 7–59). The cementum is formed by numerous plump cementoblasts (Figs. 7–63 and 7–64). The intimate relationship of the lesion to the tooth (i.e., attached to and replacing root) is an important diagnostic sign. The tooth is sacrificed with removal of this nonrecurring lesion.

■ Periapical Cemento-Osseous Dysplasia

This is a common reactive/dysplastic process of unknown etiology that occurs at the apices of vital mandibular teeth (especially incisors), predominantly in middle-aged, and often black, women (Fig. 7–60). Because it is diagnostic radiographically and needs no treatment, it is infrequently biopsied. It is occasionally seen at the apex of posterior teeth, where it is more likely to be confused with periapical inflammatory disease (Fig. 7–61). This asymptomatic process passes through several stages: lucent, mixed lucent-opaque, and opaque. No treatment is necessary because the process is self-limited.

Microscopically, periapical cemento-osseous dysplasia appears as a benign fibro-osseous lesion (Figs. 7–65 and 7–68). A benign fibroblastic matrix contains a heterogeneous distribution of new bone trabeculae and cementum-type material. Inflammatory cells are scant.

■ Florid Osseous Dysplasia

This is believed to be an exuberant form of periapical cemento-osseous dysplasia. In addition to periapical lesions, this condition may affect the entire jaw (usually mandible) (Fig. 7–62). Traumatic bone cysts may be seen in association with this process. Florid osseous dysplasia is often biopsied because of its remarkable radiographic picture. It may also be associated with traumatic bone cysts.

Florid osseous dysplasia appears microscopically as a benign fibro-osseous lesion. Bony islands and trabeculae are seen in a bland connective tissue matrix (Figs. 7–69 and 7–70). Inflammatory cells are scant. Clinical correlation is necessary to make a definitive diagnosis. Unfortunately, florid osseous dysplasia may become secondarily infected, superimposing a chronic osteomyelitis on the process and making diagnosis more difficult. Florid osseous dysplasia, like its periapical cousin, requires no treatment, unless secondarily infected.

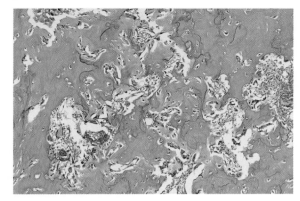

FIG. 7–63. Cementoblastoma

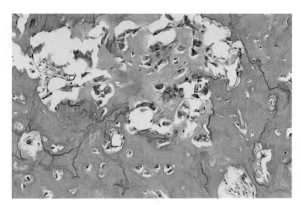

FIG. 7–64. High magnification of Figure 7–63

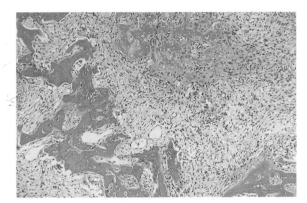

FIG. 7–65. Periapical cemento-osseous dysplasia

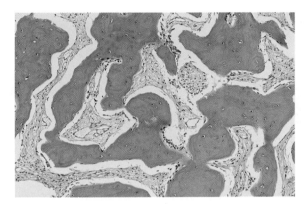

FIG. 7–66. Periapical cemento-osseous dysplasia

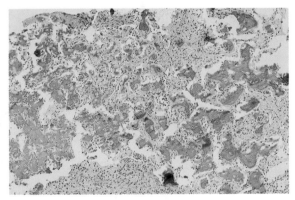

FIG. 7–67. Periapical cemento-osseous dysplasia

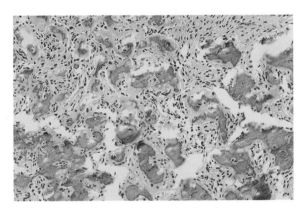

FIG. 7–68. Periapical cemento-osseous dysplasia

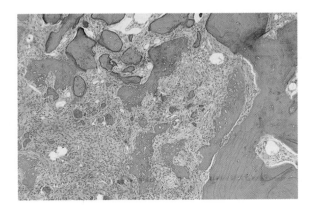

FIG. 7–69. Florid osseous dysplasia

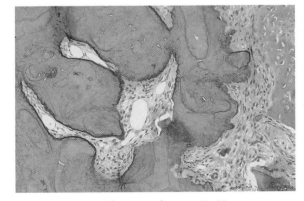

FIG. 7–70. High magnification of Figure 7–69

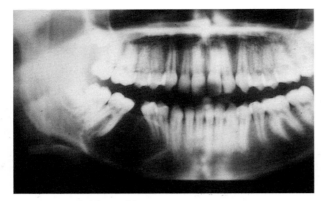

FIG. 7–71. Ameloblastic fibroma

■ Ameloblastic Fibroma

This is a mixed odontogenic tumor composed of only soft tissues. It is seen in teenagers and only rarely over the age of 30. It is a well-circumscribed radiolucent tumor (Fig. 7–71), except when an odontoma is also present (see below). This tumor has a predilection for the posterior jaws. It is generally curetted along a cleavage plane, and recurrence is infrequent.

Microscopically, ameloblastic fibroma has a characteristic composition of lobular myxoid connective tissue with strands of odontogenic epithelium (Figs. 7–75 and 7–76). Diagnosis must be made in the correct clinical context, because hyperplastic follicular sacs with numerous rests occasionally exhibit a similar appearance. Some tumors may have an attached odontoma, prompting the diagnosis of *ameloblastic fibro-odontoma* (Fig. 7–72).

Rarely seen is a lesion called *ameloblastic fibrosarcoma*, in which the connective tissue component has histologic features of a fibrosarcoma (Figs. 7–77 and 7–78). This lesion, seen at an older age, is regarded as a locally aggressive lesion.

■ Odontoma

Odontoma is a relatively common mixed odontogenic hamartoma that is composed of dental hard tissues. If miniature teeth can be recognized, the lesion is called *compound odontoma* (Fig. 7–73); if not, it is called *complex odontoma* (Figs. 7–74, 7–79, 7–80). Children and teenagers are most commonly affected. The lesions contain dentin, enamel, and frequently remnants of the cells that form them. Except for rare large complex lesions, odontomas are simply space-occupying lesions that, at worst, block eruption of teeth. Removal is recommended.

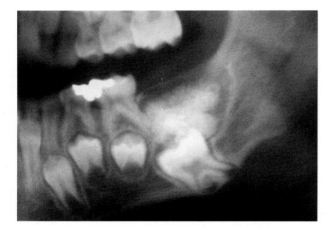

FIG. 7–72. Ameloblastic fibro-odontoma

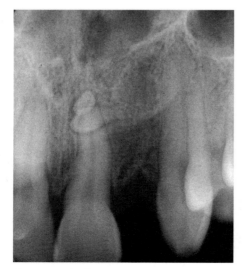

FIG. 7–73. Compound odontoma

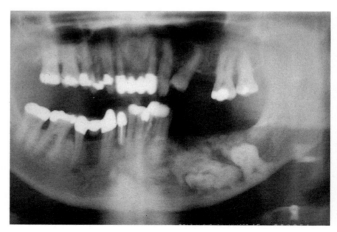

FIG. 7–74. Complex odontoma

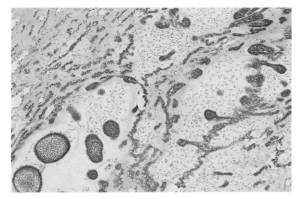

FIG. 7-75. Ameloblastic fibroma

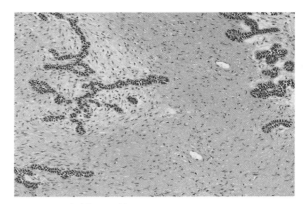

FIG. 7-76. Ameloblastic fibroma

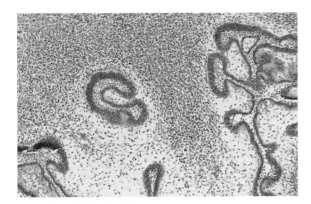

FIG. 7-77. Ameloblastic fibrosarcoma

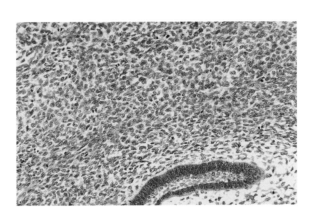

FIG. 7-78. High magnification of Figure 7-77

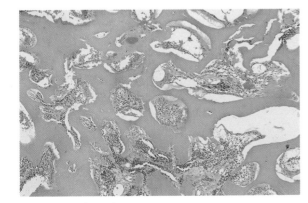

FIG. 7-79. Complex odontoma

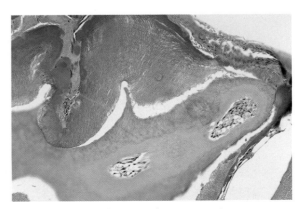

FIG. 7-80. High magnification of Figure 7-79

Giant Cell Lesions of the Jaws

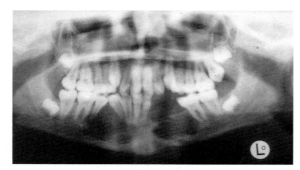

FIG. 8–1. CGCG of mandible

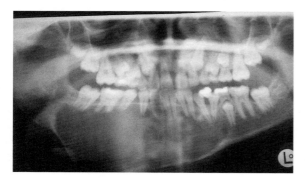

FIG. 8–2. CGCG of mandible

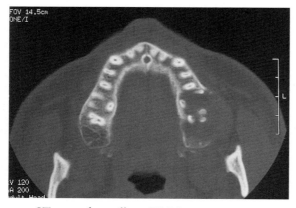

FIG. 8–3. CT scan of maxillary CGCG

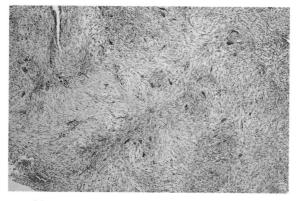

FIG. 8–4. Heterogeneous pattern, CGCG

■ Central Giant Cell Granuloma

Central giant cell granuloma (CGCG) appears to be a lesion that is unique to the jaws, although so-called giant cell reaction of the hands and feet shares many features. CGCG was formerly regarded as a reparative process and was accordingly called central giant cell *reparative* granuloma. While many investigators believe that it should be classified as a reactive lesion, numerous documented aggressive and recurrent cases suggest that it may occasionally behave more like a neoplasm. There is currently no way to predict which lesions will behave badly.

ETIOLOGY AND PATHOGENESIS

CGCG appears to be a tumor in which osteoclasts or their precursors are recruited into a predominantly fibroblastic field. The fibroblasts are in cell cycle and may produce cytokines/ growth factors that support tumor growth.

CLINICAL FEATURES

CGCGs occur typically in the second and third decades (mean age of approximately 25 years). Recurrences are more likely in children than adults. Females are more frequently affected than males. CGCG has a predilection for the mandible, especially the body and anterior portions of the jaw. The lesion is radiolucent and usually multilocular (Figs. 8–1 to 8–3). Resorption and/or movement of teeth may be seen, and penetration of jaw cortex may occur. Most patients are asymptomatic, although pain or paresthesia may be a presenting complaint, particularly in aggressive lesions.

MICROSCOPIC FEATURES

Histologically, a number of patterns may be seen (Figs. 8–4 to 8–6). The stroma may be fibrotic and/or myxoid in appearance. New bone may be present, especially at the periphery of the lesion. Recent and old hemorrhage is typically found. Necrosis is not evident. The dominant stromal cells are fibroblastic in origin (Fig. 8–7). They may be particularly numerous, and mitotic figures may be frequently seen. Giant cells (CD68-positive, Fig. 8–8) vary in size, shape, and number. Also, nuclei in the giant cells may be few to numerous, and their distribution may be diffuse or patchy.

The aggressive, recurrent giant cell tumor of long bone (GCT) is generally believed to be an entity separate from CGCG (Figs. 8–9 and 8–10). Most recognize its rare occurrence in the jaws, however. Because CGCG and GCT have overlapping histopathologic features, separation of these two lesions is difficult. Some features that suggest GCT over CGCG include large giant cells, large numbers of nuclei in giant cells, central aggregation of giant cell nuclei, diffusely distributed giant cells, high stromal cellularity, and necrosis. Microscopic differential diagnosis of CGCG lookalikes include aneurysmal bone cyst, hyperparathyroidism, cherubism, and possibly well-differentiated osteosarcoma with giant cells.

TREATMENT

Surgery has been the treatment of choice. Alternative medical therapy of calcitonin injections has shown some promising results in the reduction of large lesions (Figs. 8–11 and 8–12).

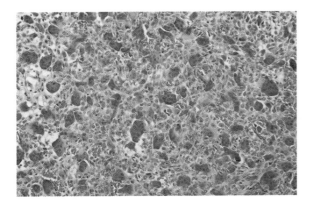

FIG. 8–5. CGCG

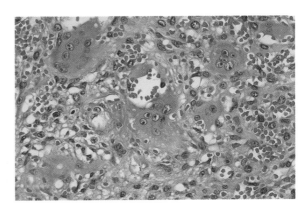

FIG. 8–6. High magnification of CGCG

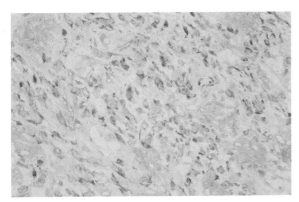

FIG. 8–7. Positive propyl-4-hydroxylase stain for CGCG fibroblasts

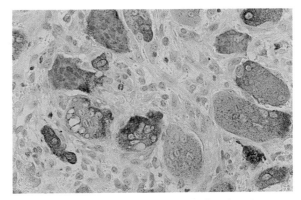

FIG. 8–8. Positive stain for macrophage-related antigen (CD68)

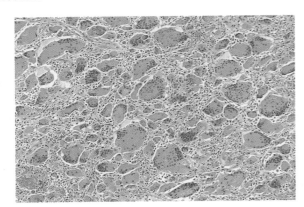

FIG. 8–9. GCT of long bones

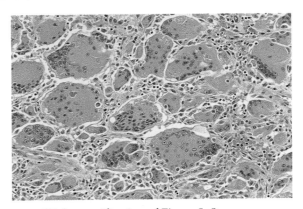

FIG. 8–10. High magnification of Figure 8–9

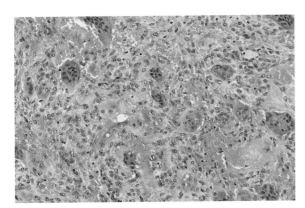

FIG. 8–11. Microscopy of CGCG in Figure 8–1

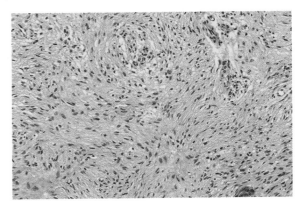

FIG. 8–12. Biopsy of CGCG in Figure 8–1 after 1 year of calcitonin Tx

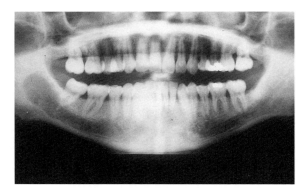

FIG. 8–13. Aneurysmal bone cyst of right mandible

■ Aneurysmal Bone Cyst

This lesion appears as a well-defined radiolucency in the jaws (Fig. 8–13). Aneurysmal bone cyst is separated from CGCG through the identification of large sinusoidal vascular channels that are not lined by endothelial cells (Fig. 8–14). Bony trabeculae, partially surrounding or circumscribing the vascular spaces, may also be present. Because clinical and radiographic features are similar to CGCG, differentiation is based primarily on microscopic features. The aneurysmal bone cyst is a reactive lesion of unknown pathogenesis, although it is thought to be related to focally altered hemodynamics. It may occur as a primary lesion or as a secondary lesion in association with a pre-existing bone lesion (e.g., fibrous dysplasia).

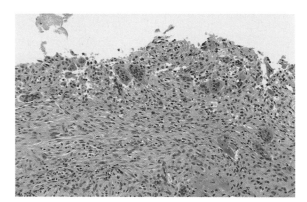

FIG. 8–14. Aneurysmal bone cyst with giant cell lining

■ Hyperparathyroidism

Hyperparathyroidism is a result of elevated blood levels of parathyroid hormone. This may be due to primary parathyroid gland disease (hyperplasia or neoplasia, most commonly adenoma) or secondary disease (hormone overproduction in response to hypocalcemia, as in renal failure).

Patients with hyperparathyroidism may have systemic signs and symptoms that include fatigue, weakness, nausea, polyuria, thirst, depression, bone pain, and evidence of bone demineralization (osteitis fibrosa cystica). Oral manifestations include multiple jaw radiolucencies (giant cell lesions) (Fig. 8–15) and loss of definition of the lamina dura around the roots of teeth (Fig. 8–16).

Elevated serum calcium and parathormone levels are indicative of hyperparathyroidism. Serum chemistry is within normal limits for patients with microscopically indistinguishable CGCG (Fig. 8–17). Because hyperparathyroidism is similar to other giant cell lesions, diagnosis is based on clinicopathologic correlation.

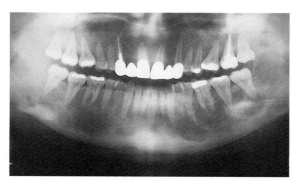

FIG. 8–15. Multiple lucencies of hyperparathyroidism

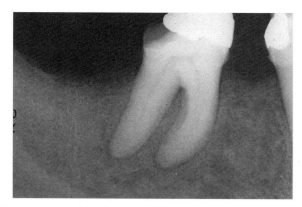

FIG. 8–16. Loss of lamina dura in hyperparathyroidism

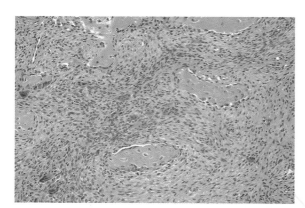

FIG. 8–17. Hyperparathyroidism with giant cell among fibroblasts

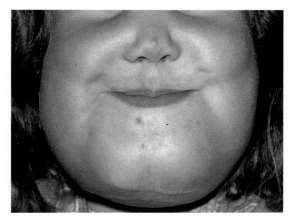

FIG. 8–18. Cherubism of maxilla and mandible

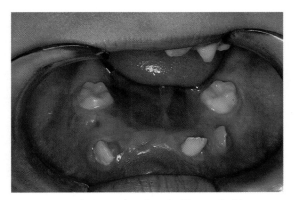

FIG. 8–19. Intraoral view of patient in Figure 8–18

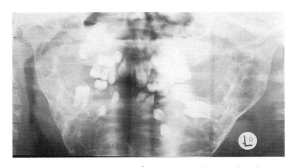

FIG. 8–20. Panoramic image of patient in Figure 8–18

■ Cherubism

Cherubism is an autosomal disorder in which multiple and nearly symmetrical giant cell lesions of the jaws appear in early childhood. It is a self-limiting disease that seems to stabilize after puberty. The designation of cherubism comes from the typical cherubic facies that these patients develop due to maxillary expansion associated with lesion growth.

CLINICAL AND RADIOGRAPHIC FEATURES

The mandibular body and ramus and posterior maxilla are most commonly affected (Figs. 8–18 and 8–19). Lesions affect either two or four quadrants. The swelling is gradual and painless. The maxillary lesion may expand to the maxillary sinuses and orbit floor. Lymphadenopathy may be evident in the cervical nodes.

Radiographically, the lesions appear as loculated radiolucencies that have been described as having a "soap bubble" appearance (Fig. 8–20). Teeth may be missing, malformed, or displaced.

MICROSCOPIC FEATURES

Cherubism is another giant cell lesion that histologically resembles the more common CGCG (Figs. 8–21 and 8–22). A distinctive perivascular cuffing of collagen may be seen around capillaries and small vessels in cherubism.

TREATMENT

Generally, once the diagnosis is confirmed microscopically, no treatment is necessary. Surgical recontouring may on occasion be needed to achieve improved cosmetic appearance and function. After puberty , the lesions should stabilize and begin to show radiographic evidence of resolution.

Separation of cherubism from CGCG should be relatively easy on clinical grounds. Lesions of cherubism are bilaterally symmetrical and may affect all four quadrants. Other family members will also be affected due to the hereditary nature of this condition.

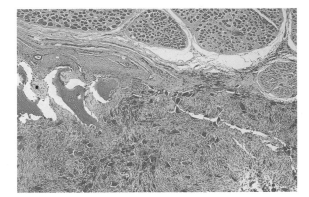

FIG. 8–21. Tissue specimen from patient in Figure 8–18

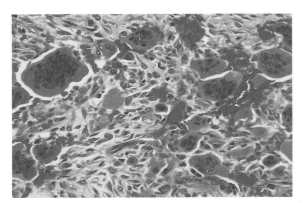

FIG. 8–22. High magnification of Figure 8–21

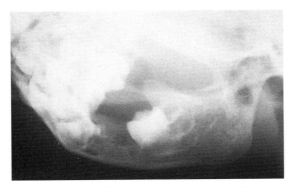

FIG. 8–23. Langerhans cell disease of posterior mandible

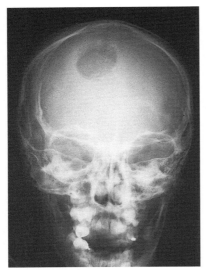

FIG. 8–24. Langerhans cell disease of skull

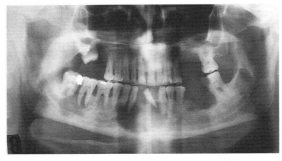

FIG. 8–25. Langerhans cell disease of mandibular alveolus

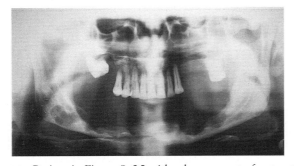

FIG. 8–26. Patient in Figure 8–25 with advancement of untreated disease

■ Langerhans Cell Disease

This condition, formerly known as *idiopathic histiocytosis* and *histiocytosis X*, is a proliferation of Langerhans cells that is difficult to classify as either a reactive or neoplastic process. It is included among the giant cell lesions for lack of a better place and because it may contain tumor giant cells.

ETIOLOGY AND PATHOGENESIS

Biologically, Langerhans cell disease seems to lie somewhere between an ideopathic reaction and a true neoplasm. While the cell of origin appears to be confirmed, the cause of its proliferation remains a mystery. It has been speculated that because Langerhans cells have the function of immune surveillance, tumor formation is related to chronic antigenic stimulation.

CLINICAL FEATURES

Three forms of this disease are recognized: acute disseminated (also known as Letterer-Siwe disease) is a lethal malignant proliferation in childhood; chronic disseminated (also known as Hand-Schuller-Christian syndrome) results in focal lesions in lymph nodes, viscera, and bones; and chronic localized (also known as eosinophilic granuloma) causes bone lesion(s) only (Figs. 8–23 and 8–24).

When the jaws are involved in this process, it is usually in the form of the solitary monostotic type (eosinophilic granuloma or chronic localized). Occasionally, multiple and polyostotic lesions and soft tissue involvement may be seen orally. There may be pain and swelling and "spontaneous" tooth loss. Lesions appear as sharply demarcated punched-out lucencies. When the alveolar process is involved, a "floating teeth" radiographic image is seen (Figs. 8–25 and 8–26).

MICROSCOPIC FEATURES

Microscopically, pale cells with a macrophage-like appearance dominate the field (Figs. 8–27 and 8–28). Multinucleated giant cells (Fig. 8–29), eosinophils, and necrosis may also be seen. When the process occurs near the apex of a tooth, it may be confused with periapical granuloma. Both processes (Langerhans cell disease and periapical granuloma) may be superimposed on each other. The normal cellular counterparts to these tumor cells are found among prickle cells in epithelium and are known as the Langerhans cells (a relative of the macrophage) (Figs. 8–31 and 8–32). Both normal Langerhans cells and tumor cells are CD1 and S-100 positive (Fig. 8–30). They are negative for macrophage antigens, such as CD68. Ultrastructure of the tumor cells shows the presence of numerous Langerhans or Birbeck granules that characterize normal Langerhans cells (Figs. 8–33 and 8–34).

TREATMENT

The rare acute disseminated form is usually fatal despite administration of chemotherapeutic drugs. The chronic disseminated form is treated with chemotherapy and/or local radiation. Surgical excision of individual lesions may also be a useful adjunct. Chronic localized disease is managed with surgical curettage and/or low-dose radiation. If there are several bone lesions, chemotherapy may be used. Although recurrences are sometimes seen, the prognosis for the typical localized disease seen in the jaws is very good.

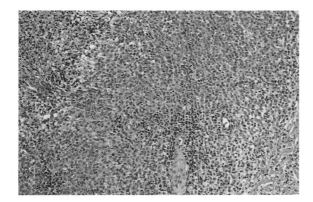

FIG. 8–27. Langerhans cell disease infiltrate

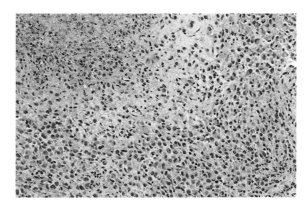

FIG. 8–28. Langerhans cell infiltrate—necrosis, top left

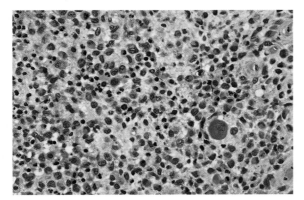

FIG. 8–29. Giant cells in Langerhans cell disease

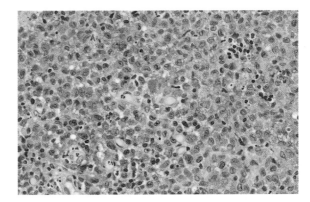

FIG. 8–30. S-100-positive stain of Langerhans cell disease

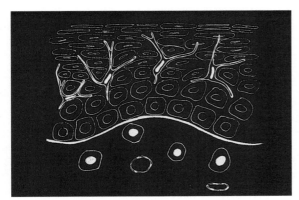

FIG. 8–31. Diagram of normal Langerhans cells in epithelium

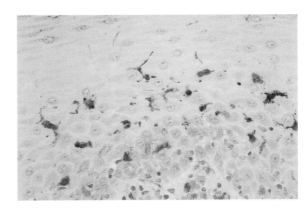

FIG. 8–32. S-100-positive stain of normal Langerhans cells

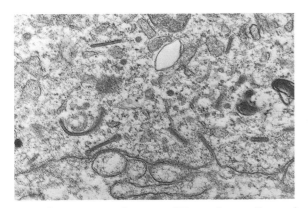

FIG. 8–33. Ultrastructure of tumor cell Langerhans cell granules

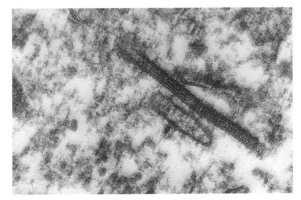

FIG. 8–34. High magnification of Figure 8–33

CHAPTER 8: Giant Cell Lesions of the Jaws

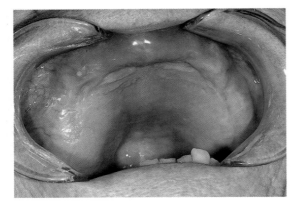

FIG. 8–35. Paget's disease of maxilla

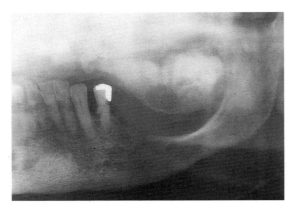

FIG. 8–36. Paget's disease of jaws

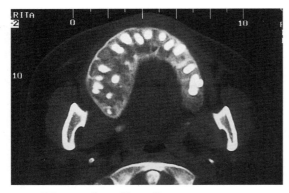

FIG. 8–37. CT scan of maxillary disease

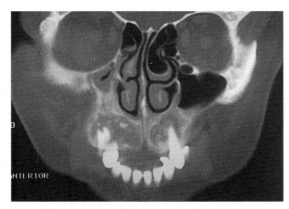

FIG. 8–38. CT scan of maxillary Paget's disease

■ Paget's Disease

Paget's disease (osteitis deformans) is a chronic condition of undetermined origin that results in uniform expansion and ossification of bones of the skeleton. Paget's bone is at risk (up to 15% of patients) for transformation to osteosarcoma. The disease is progressive and there is no cure. Therapeutic regimens are generally directed at controlling bone metabolism and pain.

ETIOLOGY AND PATHOGENESIS
Although the cause is unknown, autoimmunity, endocrine abnormality, genetic defect in connective tissue metabolism, and viral infection have all been postulated.

CLINICAL FEATURES
Paget's disease typically affects patients over the age of 50. The bones most commonly affected are the spine, femur, cranium, pelvis, and sternum. The mandible and/or the maxilla are involved in over 15% of cases. Depending on the bones involved, pain, headache, visual changes, auditory complaints, facial paralysis, vertigo, and weakness may be seen. Serum calcium and serum phosphate levels are normal. However, serum alkaline phosphatase levels are markedly elevated, reflective of the intense osteoblastic activity in the affected bone(s).

The jaws show a gradual symmetrical enlargement that is often painful (Fig. 8–35) . Edentulous patients may complain that their dentures are too tight. Dentulous patients may develop diastemas between teeth, and teeth may become loose.

Radiographically, bone patterns will be variable and are dependent on disease stage (Figs. 8–36 to 8–38). Early in the disease process, bone may appear relatively lucent. As the disease progresses, bone becomes densely opaque. In the jaws, lamina dura and periodontal membrane spaces may become obliterated. Teeth may show hypercementosis or resorption.

MICROSCOPIC FEATURES
Osteoclasts and capillaries dominate the early phase of Paget's disease. Later, numerous osteoblasts and osteoclasts are seen. Abundant reversal lines become apparent as the bone undergoes continual remodeling (Fig. 8–39). End-stage Paget's bone is densely sclerotic and exhibits a mosaic pattern that reflects the remodeling process. Very little marrow is seen.

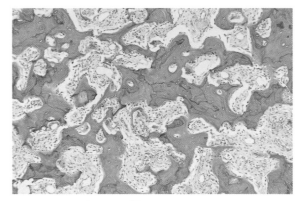

FIG. 8–39. Paget's disease of bone

CHAPTER 8: Giant Cell Lesions of the Jaws

CHAPTER 9

Fibro-Osseous Lesions of the Jaws

Ossifying Fibroma

Fibrous Dysplasia

Desmoplastic Fibroma

Osteoblastoma

Osteoma

Torus

Exostosis

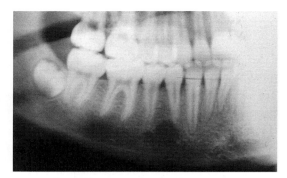

FIG. 9–1. Ossifying fibroma in body of mandible

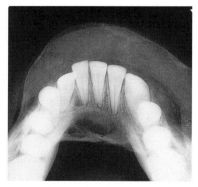

FIG. 9–2. Ossifying fibroma of anterior mandible

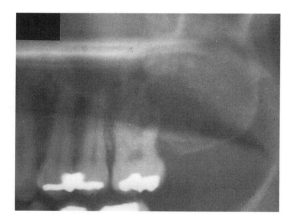

FIG. 9–3. Ossifying fibroma of posterior maxilla

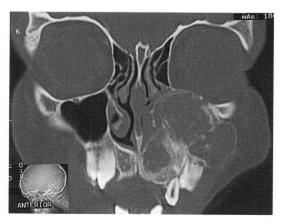

FIG. 9–4. CT scan of maxillary ossifying fibroma

■ Ossifying Fibroma

Fibro-osseous lesions are a diverse group of conditions that vary widely in clinical-radiographic presentation and biologic behavior. Because there is considerable histologic overlap within this group as well as with some odontogenic tumors, osteomyelitis, and some osteosarcomas, diagnosis from histologic features alone can be difficult. Microscopically, the lesions are composed of a fibroblastic stroma in which there is new bone formed.

Ossifying fibroma is a benign neoplasm of bone. It is essentially identical to lesions that have been designated as cementifying fibroma and cemento-ossifying fibroma. While differentiation of ossifying fibroma from fibrous dysplasia may at times be difficult, separation remains important because of differences in treatment and prognosis.

CLINICAL FEATURES

This lesion is slow-growing and has a predilection for the molar-ramus area of the jaws. It is discovered most commonly in the third and fourth decades, and females seem to be more frequently affected than males. An exceptional (and not universally accepted) variant, *juvenile ossifying fibroma*, appears a decade earlier. Lesions in this latter subgroup have also been called "active" and "aggressive" juvenile ossifying fibromas.

Unlike fibrous dysplasia, ossifying fibroma is a well-circumscribed lesion with distinct margins (Fig. 9–1). This is frequently evident radiographically as an opaque margin that surrounds these lesions. Ossifying fibroma appears as a relatively radiolucent lesion when compared to surrounding bone (Fig. 9–2). When the osseous trabeculae in the tumor are sufficiently large and calcified, opaque foci may be seen (Figs. 9–3 and 9–4).

MICROSCOPIC FEATURES

Microscopically, ossifying fibroma is sharply demarcated from surrounding resident bone. The tumor bone is seen in the form of uniform trabeculae or oval (spherical) islands (Figs. 9–5 to 9–7). Jaw lesions that contain predominately oval hard tissue islands, instead of osseous trabeculae, have been referred to as *cemento-* or *psammomatoid-ossifying fibromas* (Fig. 9–8). This segregation is essentially academic because the behaviors of these lesions are the same. Osteoblasts are usually prominent, rimming the new bone. Stromal cellularity of ossifying fibroma may be relatively high in contrast to fibrous dysplasia, and it may vary from one area to another. The stroma in the so-called juvenile ossifying fibroma is particularly cellular but still cytologically benign. The bone in these lesions appears in the form of strands or trabeculae, although psammomatoid ossicles may be evident. With time, ossifying fibromas change little microscopically (Figs. 9–9 and 9–10), although they increase in size.

TREATMENT

Because there is often a distinct fibrous connective capsule, ossifying fibroma may be enucleated. While most lesions seem to have limited growth potential, occasional lesions exhibit considerable growth with bone destruction, differences that cannot be predicted from the microscopic features. The juvenile variant is generally thought to have a greater propensity for aggressive behavior.

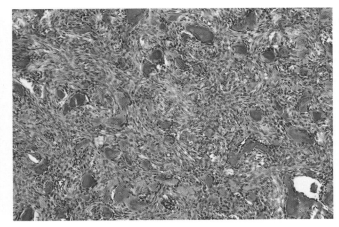

FIG. 9–5. Ossifying fibroma with new bone in fibroblastic matrix

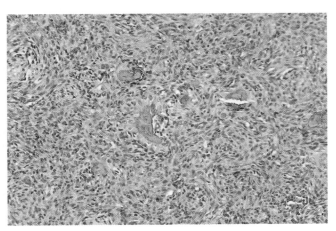

FIG. 9–6. Ossifying fibroma with small islands of new bone

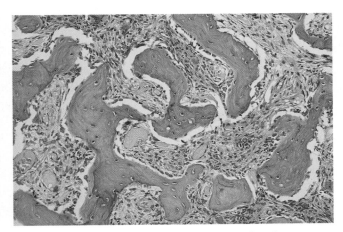

FIG. 9–7. Ossifying fibroma with new bone trabeculae

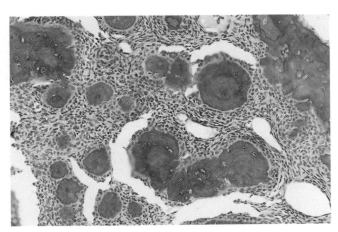

FIG. 9–8. Ossifying fibroma with psammomatoid bone

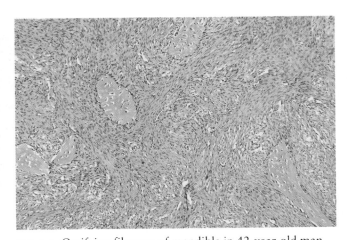

FIG. 9–9. Ossifying fibroma of mandible in 42-year-old man

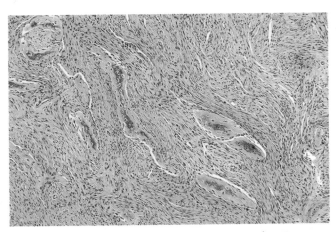

FIG. 9–10. Biopsy of untreated tumor (Fig. 9–9) after 7 years

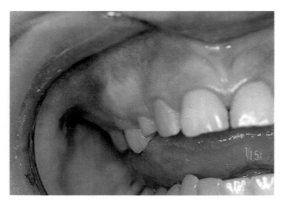

FIG. 9–11. Bony expansion of maxilla due to fibrous dysplasia

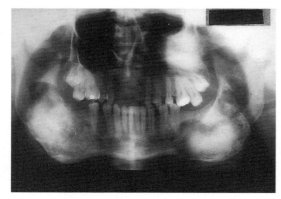

FIG. 9–12. Fibrous dysplasia of mandible and maxilla

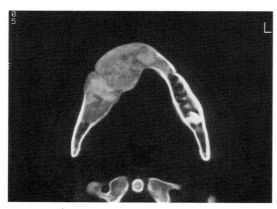

FIG. 9–13. CT scan of mandibular fibrous dysplasia

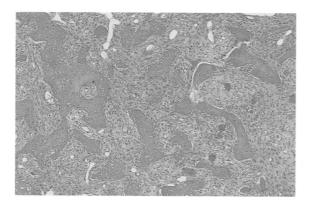

FIG. 9–14. Fibrous dysplasia of mandible

■ Fibrous Dysplasia

Fibrous dysplasia is a condition in which there is gradual replacement of normal bone by fibrous connective tissue and structurally weak fibrillar bone. The stimulus for such a change is unknown. The biologic behavior of fibrous dysplasia indicates that it does not represent a neoplastic lesion. Instead, because of its self-limited growth and apparent response to the hormonal changes of puberty, it is classified as a dysplastic process.

CLINICAL AND RADIOGRAPHIC FEATURES

Fibrous dysplasia may be limited to one bone (monostotic type) or it may involve several bones (polyostotic type). If the polyostotic type occurs in association with endocrine abnormalities, particularly precocious puberty and pigmented skin macules, it is referred to as *Albright's (McCune-Albright's) syndrome*. It is a self-limiting, slow-growing process that starts in childhood. Swelling is unilateral and asymptomatic. In the craniofacial complex, it is most commonly seen in the maxilla (Fig. 9–11) and calvarium, while in the remainder of the skeleton, it is most frequently seen in the rib, femur, and tibia. Jaw lesions may result in significant facial deformity. Involvement of the orbits, sinuses, and/or cranial ostia may cause nasal obstruction, sinusitis, headache, and hearing and visual disturbances. Outside the craniofacial complex, pain is the most common presenting symptom.

Radiographically, fibrous dysplasia has ill-defined margins and blends into surrounding bone (Figs. 9–12 and 9–13). It typically has the appearance of a diffusely radiopaque lesion, varying from characteristic "ground glass" to sclerotic. Although the affected bone may surround teeth, looseness or exfoliation is not seen. Serum laboratory values are usually within normal limits, unless the patient has extensive polyostotic disease, which may result in an elevation of serum alkaline phosphatase.

MICROSCOPIC FEATURES

Fibrous dysplasia consists of a relatively vascular and loose benign fibrous connective tissue stroma surrounding immature fibrillar or woven bony trabeculae (Fig. 9–14). The stroma generally exhibits only low to moderate cellularity. The incompletely calcified bony trabeculae show some regularity in size and are uniformly distributed throughout, gradually blending into normal surrounding bone. Osteoclasts are typically inconspicuous and osteoblasts are scant, providing an appearance to the tumor bone that has been referred to as "osseous metaplasia." As patients with fibrous dysplasia age, affected bone may show some maturation in the form of lamellations.

TREATMENT

The process usually stabilizes during puberty, persisting in a nearly quiescent state indefinitely. When treatment is necessary to alleviate unacceptable facial deformity, surgical recontouring rather than complete excision is preferred. Regrowth of surgically recontoured fibrous dysplasia is seen in approximately 25% of cases. Complete or partial excision with bone grafting has been recently used with some success. An increased risk of malignant transformation of fibrous dysplasia to sarcoma has been observed, although many sarcomas have followed therapeutic radiation of the involved bone.

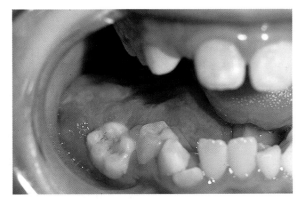

FIG. 9–15. Desmoplastic fibroma; differential included fibrosarcoma

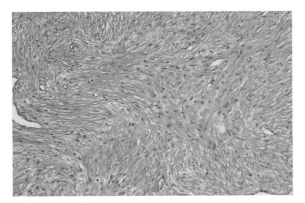

FIG. 9–16. Fascicular pattern of desmoplastic fibroma

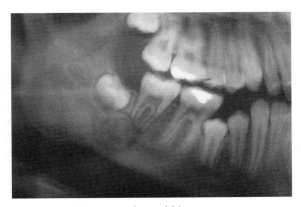

FIG. 9–17. Osteoblastoma of mandible

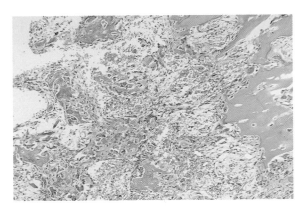

FIG. 9–18. Osteoblastoma of mandible

■ Desmoplastic Fibroma

This is a rare fibrous lesion of the jaws. It is benign but aggressive, and has a behavior similar to fibromatosis of soft tissue or low-grade fibrosarcoma (Fig. 9–15). It is seen in young adults, especially in the mandible. Radiographically, desmoplastic fibroma is lucent, with margins that may be distinct or poorly defined.

Histologically, these lesions exhibit an interlacing or fascicular growth pattern of benign fibroblasts and collagen (Fig. 9–16). They neither contain epithelial rests nor make bone. Multinucleated giant cells are also generally absent. Desmoplastic fibroma should not be confused with the more atypical and cellular central low-grade osteosarcoma.

■ Osteoblastoma

This is a benign fibro-osseous lesion that is regarded as a larger version of osteoid osteoma. It is usually seen in the vertebrae and long bones, and rarely in either jaw as a well-defined lucency or relative opacity. It is similar clinically and radiographically to ossifying fibroma (Fig. 9–17), but is frequently associated with pain, is seen in a younger age group (second decade), and affects males more often than females. Either jaw may be affected. Conservative surgical removal is recommended.

Microscopically, osteoblastoma is differentiated from ossifying fibroma by its prominent and abundant osteoblasts (Figs. 9–18 and 9–19). The stroma may be very vascular, and osteoclasts may be seen.

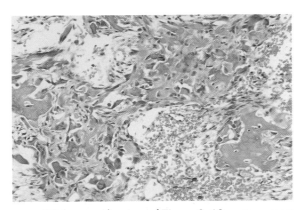

FIG. 9–19. High magnification of Figure 9–18; note numerous osteoblasts

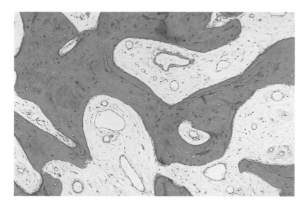

FIG. 9–20. Osteoma

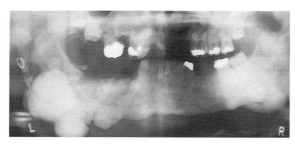

FIG. 9–21. Multiple osteomas of Gardner's syndrome

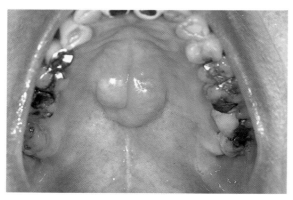

FIG. 9–22. Palatal torus

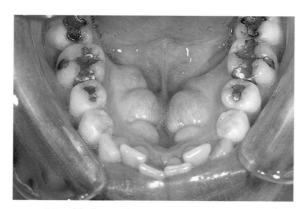

FIG. 9–23. Mandibular tori

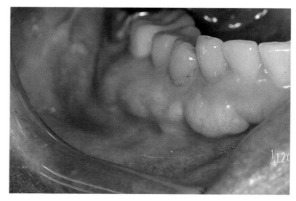

FIG. 9–24. Exostoses of mandibular buccal cortex

■ Osteoma

This is an uncommon to rare benign lesion of the jaws. It presents as a circumscribed radiodense mass that may be confused both radiographically and microscopically with common focal sclerosing osteitis. Osteomas are not microscopically distinctive, being composed simply of mature bone and small amounts of fibrous marrow (Fig. 9–20).

Osteoma is of particular significance when it occurs as part of Gardner's syndrome (multiple osteomas, intestinal polyposis, skin cysts, impacted and supernumerary teeth, odontomas) (Fig. 9–21). The gastrointestinal polyps, found in the colon and rectum, are at very high risk for malignant transformation.

■ Torus

Torus is a nodular bony protuberance of either the midline of the palate (Fig. 9–22) or the lingual mandible (Fig. 9–23). Approximately 20% of the population have maxillary tori, and 10% have mandibular tori. The cause of these lesions is unknown, although there may be an hereditary influence. They develop during the second and third decades of life. They are asymptomatic unless the surface is traumatized during mastication. Ulcers resulting from trauma may take weeks to months to heal because of the poorly vascularized subjacent bone. Microscopically, the torus is composed of dense hyperplastic cortical-type bone. Torus is diagnostic clinically and requires no treatment. Removal may occasionally be necessary for denture construction.

■ Exostosis

Exostosis is a reactive hyperplasia of buccal cortical bone (Fig. 9–24). The process is believed, in many cases, to be related to excessive or unusual occlusal forces. The cause in the remainder is unknown. The histology of exostosis is the same as torus.

Osteomyelitis

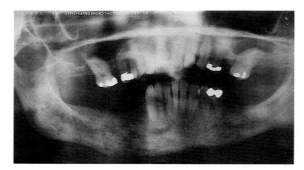

FIG. 10–1. Chronic osteomyelitis of mandible

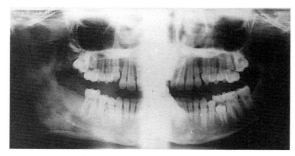

FIG. 10–2. Chronic osteomyelitis with periostitis (Garré's)

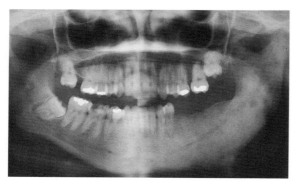

FIG. 10–3. Diffuse sclerosing osteomyelitis of mandible

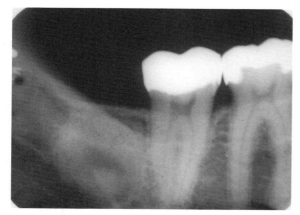

FIG. 10–4. Focal sclerosing osteitis

■ Chronic Osteomyelitis

Chronic osteomyelitis is low-grade inflammation of bone and bone marrow. This is not synonymous with infection, as microorganisms may not be the stimulus of the inflammatory process. Chronic osteomyelitis is one of several lesions that may show microscopic overlap with fibro-osseous lesions, especially ossifying fibroma and fibrous dysplasia.

CLINICAL AND RADIOGRAPHIC FEATURES
Pain and swelling are variable in chronic osteomyelitis. It is usually low-grade and intermittent. A draining sinus through usually the thinner buccal cortex is sometimes seen. The radiographic patterns for chronic osteomyelitis vary from case to case, ranging from radiolucent to mixed "moth-eaten" to opaque, depending on duration, intensity of inflammation, and individual biologic response (Fig. 10–1). Generally, a slow-progressing lesion yields more opaque material (sclerotic bone or bony scar) than a more active lesion.

MICROSCOPIC FEATURES
Inflammatory cells in chronic osteomyelitis may be quite scant, and there may be much new bone formation, giving the tissue a fibro-osseous appearance (Figs. 10–5 and 10–6). Both osteoblasts and osteoclasts may be seen. The new bony trabeculae are of irregular size and distribution, and reversal lines are likely to be evident. These features can be used to separate this condition from fibrous dysplasia and ossifying fibroma.

CLINICOPATHOLOGIC SUBTYPES
Chronic osteomyelitis with periostitis (Garré's osteomyelitis)—In the more active lesions, the bony inflammatory process may extend to involve the periosteum, resulting in peripheral expansion of the mandible, which characterizes Garré's osteomyelitis. Radiographically, this is viewed as concentric opaque layers, representing the several stages of cortex expansion (Fig. 10–2). This type of osteomyelitis may mimic fibrous dysplasia both clinically and microscopically (Figs. 10–7 and 10–8). Garré's osteomyelitis has a predilection for children and young adults and is most often related to extension of bacteria-associated pulpal and periapical inflammation. Trauma and periodontal disease are also potential causes.

Diffuse sclerosing osteomyelitis—The cause of this uncommon form of bone inflammation is often not obvious, but some cases appear to be related to low-grade bacterial infection through the periodontal membrane. It is typically seen in the mandible and seems to have a predilection for middle-aged black women. Radiographs show a dense generalized opacification of the entire jaw (Fig. 10–3). Low-level pain is also seen. It may be confused with florid osseous dysplasia because of overlapping clinical-microscopic features (Fig. 10–9). Conservative treatment is recommended, as aggressive surgery may worsen the condition.

Focal sclerosing osteitis (bony scar, condensing osteitis)—This is a common focal bone opacification seen in relationship to low-grade inflammation at the apex of teeth with chronic pulpitis. It also is seen after healing of an extraction socket or around an expanding intrabony lesion (Fig. 10–4). Microscopically, dense mature bone is seen (Fig. 10–10). Idiopathic lesions may also be seen and may be designated as *focal osteosclerosis* or *focal osteopetrosis*.

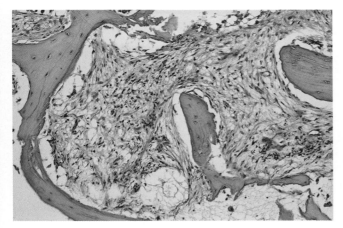

FIG. 10–5. Chronic osteomyelitis

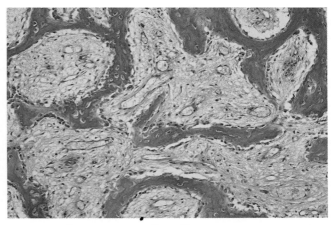

FIG. 10–6. Chronic osteomyelitis (fibro-osseous appearance)

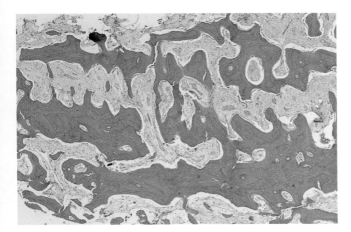

FIG. 10–7. Cortical redundancy in periostitis of Garré's

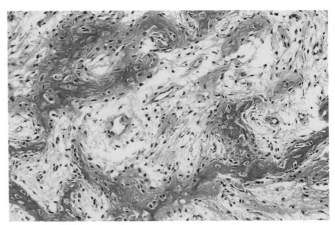

FIG. 10–8. Garré's osteomyelitis (fibro-osseous appearance)

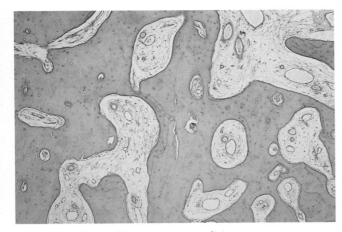

FIG. 10–9. Diffuse sclerosing osteomyelitis

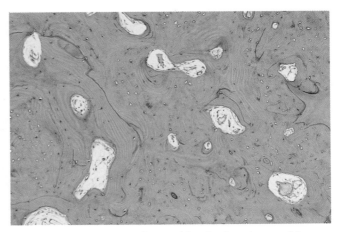

FIG. 10–10. Dense mature bone of focal sclerosing osteitis

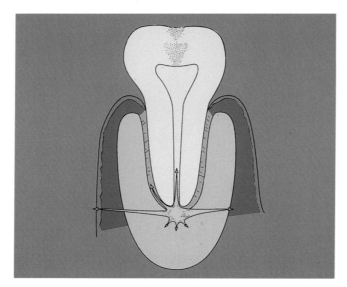

FIG. 10–11. Potential spread of pus from periapical abscess

■ Acute Osteomyelitis

Acute inflammation of maxillary or mandibular bone and bone marrow results most commonly from extension of a periapical abscess associated with a necrotic dental pulp. Physical injury (e.g., jaw fracture) is the second most common cause. Infection with bacteria is a frequent complicating factor.

Because of the intense exudation of plasma fluids and blood cells, pain is a primary feature of this bony encased inflammatory response. Pyrexia, painful lymphadenopathy, and leukocytosis are also typically associated with acute osteomyelitis of the jaws. Paresthesia of the lower lip may be present in some cases, depending on the relationship to the mandibular nerve. Because of the rapidity with which this develops, radiographic changes are minimal.

Pus (neutrophils and necrotic debris), which dominates the microscopic picture, seeks the path of least resistance (Fig. 10–11). Sequestra can often be identified in established lesions. Culture of the lesion is important for diagnosis of infection, and sensitivity testing is essential for prescribing the appropriate antibiotic.

■ Sequelae of Acute Osteomyelitis

The increasing intrabony pressure associated with the pus that characterizes this process may produce additional clinical signs in the oral mucosa, skin, or surrounding bone (Fig. 10–12). Soft tissue extension may lead to a focus of pus (abscess) or diffuse spread of pus (cellulitis). A gingival abscess associated with a periapical or periodontal abscess is known as a parulis. Sinus tracts may be seen in mucosa or skin from which pus drains until the condition is treated (Figs. 10–13 and 10–14). If drainage is achieved either surgically or by the pressure itself, symptoms are markedly relieved. Extension to the cavernous sinus may lead to a life-threatening thrombosis of this venous structure.

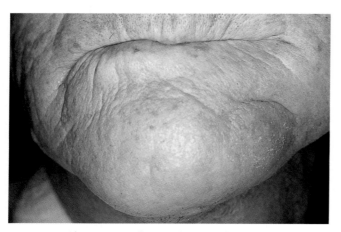

FIG. 10–12. Chronic jaw abscess about to drain through skin

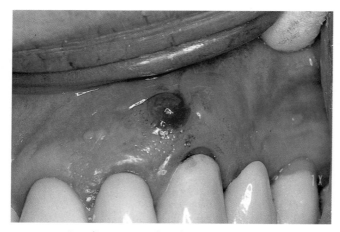

FIG. 10–13. Parulis associated with nonvital tooth

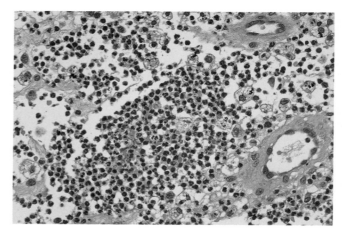

FIG. 10–14. Focus of pus in parulis

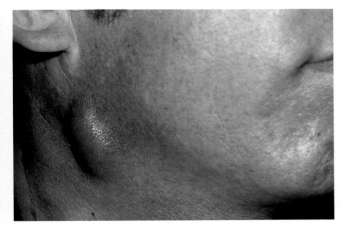

FIG. 10–15. Cervical-facial actinomycosis

■ Actinomycosis

ETIOLOGY AND PATHOGENESIS

This is a chronic infection by a microaerophilic gram-positive bacterium, *Actinomyces israelii,* and other species. This micro-organism is part of the normal oral flora and may become pathogenic when implanted in bone or soft tissue. Jaw fracture, surgical removal of a tooth, or an open root canal may be causative events. Rarely, peri-odontal disease may contribute to periodontal actinomycosis.

CLINICAL FEATURES

In the head and neck, this disease is often called cervical-facial actinomycosis because it typically presents as pain and swelling of the mandible with one or more cutaneous draining sinuses (Fig. 10–15). Pus from the lesion may contain yellow colonies of the micro-organism ("sulfur granules") (Fig. 10–16).

MICROSCOPIC FEATURES

Colonies of micro-organisms are surrounded by pus and chronically inflamed connective tissue. The colonies are mats of radiating and branching filamentous bacillary structures (Fig. 10–17). The organism is gram-positive (Fig. 10–18).

TREATMENT

Penicillin is the drug of choice for the treatment of actinomycosis. It is usually delivered in relatively high doses over an extended period of time. Surgical débridement of necrotic tissue may also assist the healing process.

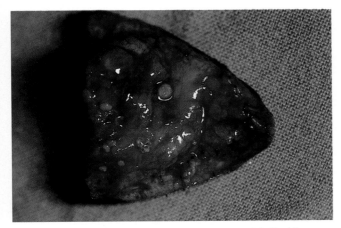

FIG. 10–16. Subcutaneous tissue (Fig. 10–15) with "sulfur granules"

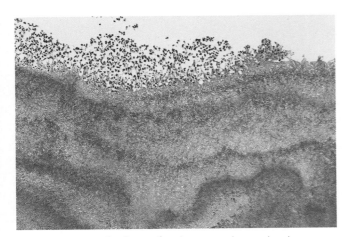

FIG. 10–17. Part of colony of actinomyces in pus (top)

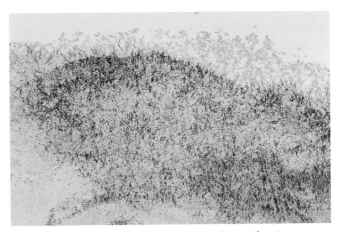

FIG. 10–18. Gram-positive filaments in colony of actinomyces

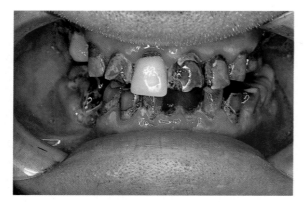

FIG. 10–19. Caries associated with radiation-induced xerostomia

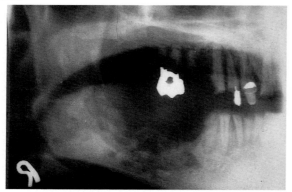

FIG. 10–20. Osteoradionecrosis eventually occurred in the patient in Figure 10–19.

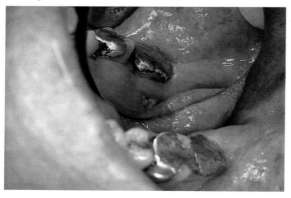

FIG. 10–21. Sequestrum from lingual mandible in radiation patient

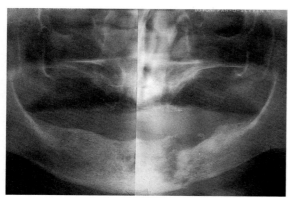

FIG. 10–22. Near pathologic fracture in radiation patient

■ Osteoradionecrosis

Therapeutic radiation for the treatment of head and neck malignancies at levels above 60 Gy has some immediate and long-term serious side effects. Occult damage, in the form of osteocyte death and vascular sclerosis, occurs in bone in the radiation path and can potentially contribute to osteoradionecrosis at a later date.

CLINICAL FEATURES

Some of the radiation side effects that are temporary and improve or disappear with time are mucosal ulcers, dysgeusia, candidiasis, and dermatitis. Permanent effects include xerostomia, increased risk for dental caries (Fig. 10–19), potential for osteonecrosis (Fig. 10–20), alopecia, epithelial atrophy, and telangiectasias.

Jaw bone that has received radiation to 60 Gy or more is susceptible to infection and has a reduced capacity for response to injury. Repair after trauma may be remarkably delayed or absent, leading to bone necrosis (osteoradionecrosis) (Fig. 10–21). Pathologic fracture may occur (Figs. 10–22 and 10–23), and sequestration of significant amounts of bone is possible. The greater the radiation level, the greater the risk. The events that may precipitate osteoradionecrosis include tooth extraction, periodontal disease, and periapical abscess. How much bone is lost due to necrosis is dependent upon radiation level, patient resistance to secondary infection, and clinical management.

TREATMENT

Conservative treatment is the general rule for postradiation treatment. An aggressive surgical approach may worsen the process. Careful débridement and antibiotics are sound approaches. Tooth extraction is best avoided unless there is compelling reason to do so, in which case the use of a relatively atraumatic procedure and antibiotics is advised. Hyperbaric oxygen has been advocated as an adjunct for the healing of osteoradionecrosis. While this may have value in selected cases, there are some possible complications (stimulation of residual neoplasm) and barriers (machine availability, cost, and patient acceptance) to this approach.

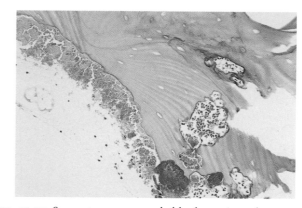

FIG. 10–23. Sequestrum surrounded by bacteria and pus

Malignancies of the Jaws

CHAPTER 12

Teeth and Periodontium

Gingivitis

Periodontitis

Scleroderma

Cleidocranial Dysplasia

Supernumerary Teeth

Fusion

Gemination

Anodontia

Taurodontism

Dens Invaginatus

Dens Evaginatus

Attrition

Abrasion

Erosion

Environmental Enamel Hypoplasia

Fluorosis

Tetracycline Stain

Amelogenesis Imperfecta

Dentinogenesis Imperfecta

Dentin Dysplasia

Regional Odontodysplasia

Internal Resorption

External Resorption

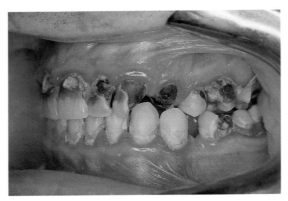

FIG. 12–1. Plaque-associated gingivitis and gross caries

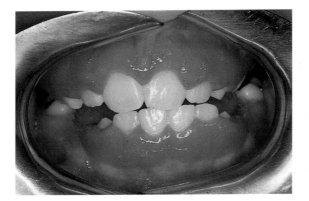

FIG. 12–2. Contact hypersensitivity (component of chewing gum)

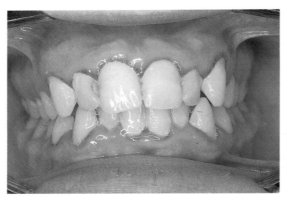

FIG. 12–3. Plaque-associated (marginal) gingivitis

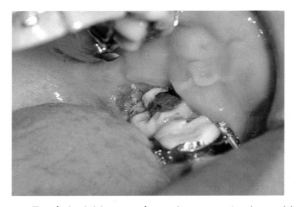

FIG. 12–4. Focal gingivitis around erupting crown (pericoronitis)

■ Gingivitis

Inflammation of the gingiva, or gingivitis, is a common condition that is directly related to the effects of dental plaque formation (Fig. 12–1). Untreated gingivitis is believed to contribute to the development of inflammation of the periodontal ligament or periodontitis, the major cause of tooth loss in adults. Inflammatory diseases of the gingiva can be subclassified into simple gingivitis, hyperplastic gingivitis, and acute necrotizing gingivitis. Noninflammatory diseases that affect gingiva and occasionally mimic it because of associated redness include mucous membrane pemphigoid, pemphigus, lichen planus, chronic lupus erythematosus, and contact hypersensitivity (Fig. 12–2).

ETIOLOGY AND PATHOGENESIS

Gingival inflammation follows the accumulation of bacterial colonized plaque on an adjacent tooth surface. The products of the mixed bacterial aggregates result in the recruitment and retention of acute (neutrophils) and chronic (lymphocytes and macrophages) inflammatory cells to the site. The process is sustained by both bacterial products and inflammatory cell cytokines/chemokines.

Dental plaque formation is a complex and dynamic process. It is composed of a cohesive matrix that holds an exuberant mixed bacterial population that varies with time, and may differ from one tooth surface to another as well as from one patient to another. Several bacterial types have been identified as being more important than others in the pathogenesis of gingivitis. Calcified dental plaque (calculus) may act as a physical irritant, but more importantly it acts as a locus for bacterial attachment and proliferation.

CLINICAL FEATURES

With the onset of inflammation, gingiva shows changes in color (red-blue), form (blunted marginal gingiva and interdental papillae), and density (spongy) (see Fig. 12–1). Gingiva bleeds easily on gentle probing of the gingival sulcus. The process is typically painless. An exudate (also known as gingival fluid) that is part of any inflammatory process can be demonstrated within the gingival sulcus. The term "marginal gingivitis" is sometimes used when inflammation is focused at the gingival margin (Fig. 12–3). Focal gingivitis may be associated with a foreign body in the gingival sulcus or trauma (Fig. 12–4). Reversal of gingivitis can be achieved by elimination and control of plaque.

Hyperplastic gingivitis is gingival inflammation in which excessive repair (hyperplastic granulation tissue and scar) has occurred (Figs. 12–5 and 12–6) (see Fibrous Lesions, Chap. 4). Acute necrotizing ulcerative gingivitis presents as gingival ulcers with overgrowth of fusiform and spirochete bacteria in debilitated patients (Figs. 12–7 and 12–8) (see Reactive Lesions, Chap. 1).

MICROSCOPIC FEATURES

Gingivitis appears as hyperemia with variable numbers of acute and chronic inflammatory cell infiltrates. Frequently plasma cells dominate, indicating marked focal stimulation of the humoral immune system. The inflammatory cells are usually focused on the sulcular side of the gingiva (adjacent to plaque) (Fig.12–9). Epithelium is often hyperplastic (Fig. 12–10), and the sulcus is sometimes ulcerated. Granulation tissue and fibrous repair become evident with time.

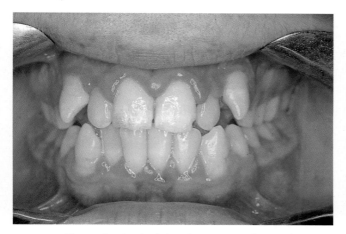

FIG. 12–5. Hyperplastic gingivitis (hormone-influenced)

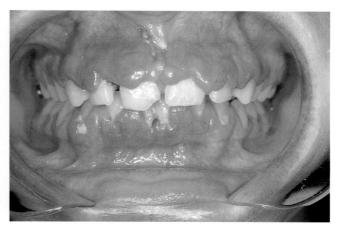

FIG. 12–6. Hyperplastic gingivitis (leukemia patient)

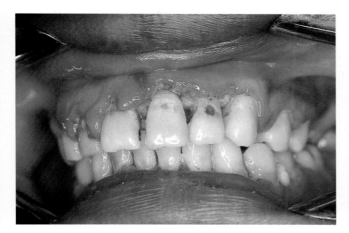

FIG. 12–7. Acute ulcerative necrotizing gingivitis

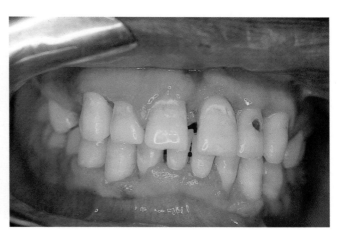

FIG. 12–8. Treated patient (Fig. 12–7) with residual defects

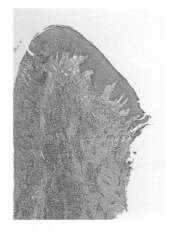

FIG. 12–9. Chronic gingivitis

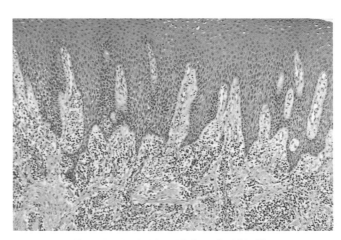

FIG. 12–10. Chronic gingivitis with lymphoid infiltrate

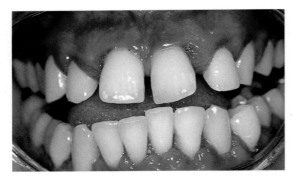

FIG. 12–11. Clinical appearance of patient with periodontitis

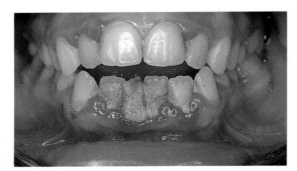

FIG. 12–12. Gingivitis and periodontitis

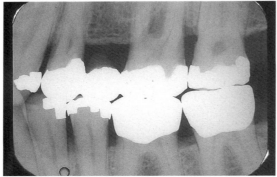

FIG. 12–13. "Horizontal" bone loss in periodontitis

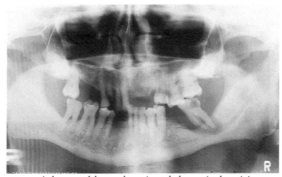

FIG. 12–14. Advanced bone loss in adult periodontitis

■ Periodontitis

Periodontitis is the most common dental disease of adults and, if left untreated, results in tooth loss. It is a complex, chronic inflammatory process that results in destruction of the structures that support teeth, namely the periodontal ligament and the alveolar bone into which it is inserted. In addition to adult periodontitis, there are several rare subtypes that may be seen in children and young adults known collectively as early-onset periodontitis (prepubertal, juvenile, or rapidly progressive periodontitis). In addition to the etiologic factors discussed below, patients with early-onset periodontitis may have an underlying immunologic or neutrophil defect.

ETIOLOGY AND PATHOGENESIS
Periodontitis is believed to be preceded by gingivitis, although some cases may show minimal signs of gingival inflammation. Pathogenic plaque—that is, plaque that supports the growth of many recognized periodontal pathogens (e.g., *Porphyromonas gingivalis*, *Actinobacillus actinomycetemcomitans*, *Treponema denticola*)—is the means by which this disease is initiated and sustained. Periodontal tissue loss is believed to be due to the effects of products of the bacteria in subgingival plaque (and calcified plaque [calculus]) as well as mediators liberated by recruited inflammatory cells. The focally released cytokines, chemokines, and proteinases cause lysis of collagen and altered function of resident fibroblasts, osteocytes, and keratinocytes.

CLINICAL FEATURES
The hallmark of periodontitis is loss of alveolar bone and associated periodontal ligament (Figs. 12–11 through 12–14). The periodontal pocket that results from this process appears as the epithelial attachment migrates apically along the tooth root. Diagnosis of periodontitis is made by clinical measurement of the coronal position of periodontal ligament (and pocket depth, Fig. 12–15) and radiographic assessment of bone loss. In generalized adult periodontitis, bone loss is uniformly "horizontal." Focal sites of bone loss may be seen in association with local conditions that support plaque retention (Fig. 12–16) and in early-onset periodontitis, such as juvenile periodontitis (Fig. 12–17). Evaluation of gingival color and architecture, gingival bleeding on probing, and tooth mobility are also of value in diagnosis. A complication of the periodontal pocket is abscess formation (Fig. 12–18).

Some systemic diseases may predispose a patient to or enhance periodontitis. These include Papillon-Lefevre syndrome, diabetes mellitus, trisomy 21, and AIDS.

MICROSCOPIC FEATURES
Alveolar bone is reduced in height and is blunted or concave due to osteoclastic resorption. The coronal end of the epithelial attachment is below the normal location at the cemento–enamel junction, reflecting the loss of periodontal ligament and alveolar bone (Figs. 12–19 and 12–20). The periodontal pocket established by this process is lined by hyperplastic nonkeratinized epithelium or ulcer. Well-vascularized connective tissue with an intense lymphocyte and plasma cell infiltrate is characteristically found subjacent to the pocket epithelium. Bacterial colonies, found in subgingival plaque, may also be evident on the pocket epithelium.

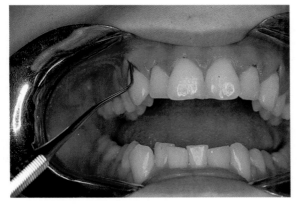

FIG. 12–15. Probe in periodontal pocket

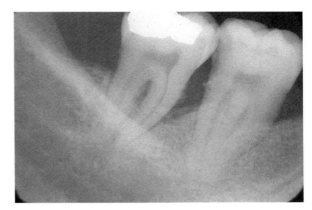

FIG. 12–16. Focal advanced bone loss

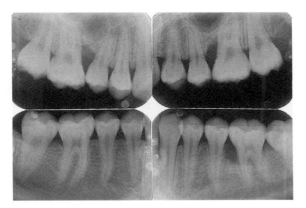

FIG. 12–17. Focal bone loss in juvenile periodontitis

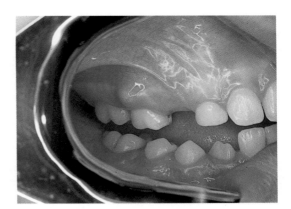

FIG. 12–18. Abscess within periodontal pocket

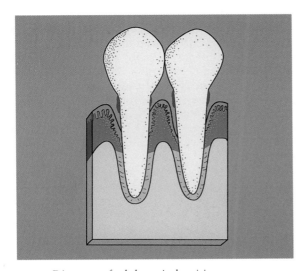

FIG. 12–19. Diagram of adult periodontitis

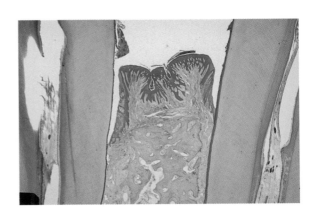

FIG. 12–20. Interdental tissue loss in periodontitis

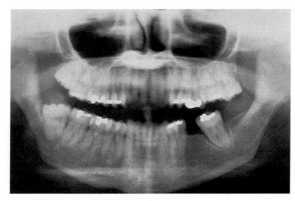

FIG. 12–21. Scleroderma—resorption of posterior mandible

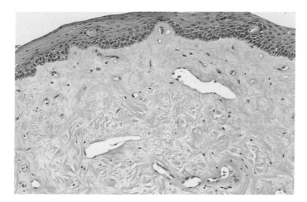

FIG. 12–22. Sclerosis of submucosa in scleroderma

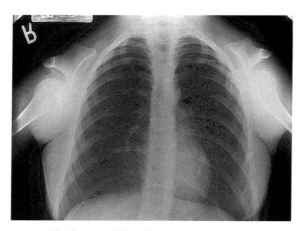

FIG. 12–23. Cleidocranial dysplasia—hypoplasia of clavicles

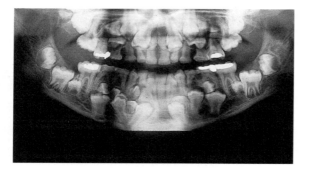

FIG. 12–24. Supernumerary teeth in cleidocranial dysplasia

■ Scleroderma

Scleroderma is a disease that can occur as a focal and potentially disfiguring lesion, or as a systemic, possibly life-threatening condition. Focal or localized scleroderma is predominately a skin phenomenon that is rarely seen in the oral mucosa. The systemic form affects many vital organs, including oral and perioral tissues, and eventually causes serious organ dysfunction through generalized fibrosis.

Scleroderma is regarded as an autoimmune disease in which there is a progressive and generalized collagenization. Both the humoral and cell-mediated immune systems appear to be involved in the pathogenesis of systemic scleroderma. Cytokines and growth factors seem to be involved in the generalized stimulation of fibroblasts. Vessel obliteration follows the collagenization of vital tissues. A fatal outcome involves compromise of the gastrointestinal tract, lungs, kidney, and/or heart. There is no satisfactory therapy for complete or adequate control of this disease.

Cutaneous manifestations of systemic scleroderma include tightening of the skin and binding to surrounding structures. The face takes on a masklike appearance, and telangiectases appear. The oral orifice becomes constricted, making access to the dentition difficult. Intraoral manifestations may be of diagnostic importance when present. The two most notable are the uniform widening of the periodontal membrane space around the roots of all teeth, and the resorption of the posterior of the mandible, best seen on Panoramic films (Fig. 12–21).

Microscopically, the submucosa becomes hypercollagenized and takes on a hyalinized appearance (Fig. 12–22). Fibroblasts and inflammatory cells are sparse. The adventitia around vessels and the subepithelial lamina propria become obliterated because of fibrosis. The above changes are common to other organs, with the additional problem of parenchymal loss and eventual organ dysfunction.

■ Cleidocranial Dysplasia

Hypoplasia/aplasia of the clavicles (Fig. 12–23), craniofacial abnormalities, and supernumerary and delayed tooth eruption make up this inherited syndrome. An enlarged calvarium results in parietal and frontal bossing. Hypoplasia of the facial bones shortens the face and gives the nose a broad flat base. Hypertelorism may also be present. Clavicular deficiency results in a characteristic appearance of a long neck and narrow drooped shoulders.

Maxillary hypoplasia provides a prognathic appearance. The palate is high-arched and narrow, and may be the site of hard and/or soft tissue clefts. Delayed or failed eruption of teeth has been associated with lack of cementum formation, particularly in relation to the permanent dentition. Supernumerary teeth are most commonly seen in the premolar region (Fig. 12–24). Significant malocclusion results from these bony and dental abnormalities.

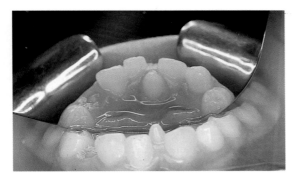

FIG. 12–25. Erupted supernumerary mesiodens

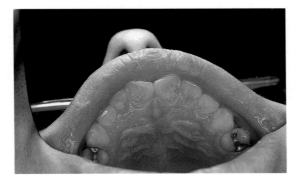

FIG. 12–26. Supernumerary incisors

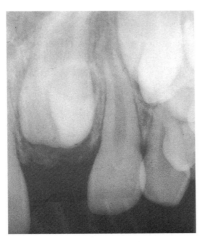

FIG. 12–27. Supernumerary tooth blocking eruption of central incisor

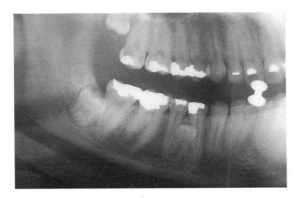

FIG. 12–28. Supernumerary premolar and molar

■ Supernumerary Teeth

Extra or supernumerary teeth in the jaws are an uncommon phenomenon that result from continued proliferation of the dental lamina for no known reason. If the dental lamina continues to differentiate after such a proliferation, a third tooth germ appears in this locus, resulting in another fully matured tooth or possibly a smaller rudimentary form. Most supernumerary teeth are the result of isolated developmental events, but some are hereditary, seen in association with *cleidocranial dysplasia* and *Gardner's syndrome* (jaw osteomas, supernumerary teeth, and malignant intestinal polyposis).

Supernumerary teeth are more commonly seen in the permanent dentition than the primary dentition, and more commonly in the maxilla than the mandible (Figs. 12–25 through 12–28). The specific sites where these teeth are found are the midline of the jaws (so-called *mesiodens*) and posterior to the maxillary molars (so-called fourth molar or *paramolar*). These teeth are of significance because they occupy valuable space in the jaws. They may block eruption of other teeth, and they may cause malalignment of teeth. They may occasionally erupt and be nonfunctional or cosmetically objectionable.

Supernumerary teeth that appear at the time of birth are known as *natal teeth*. These should not be confused with prematurely erupted deciduous teeth or soft tissue gingival cysts of the dental lamina.

After the loss of the permanent dentition, impacted supernumerary teeth may surface because of resorption of the alveolar ridge, producing what has been called a "postpermanent dentition."

Radiographic differential diagnosis of a supernumerary tooth would include other opaque lesions such as odontoma, focal sclerosing osteitis, and osteoma. Separation of some compound odontomas from supernumerary teeth is academic (Fig. 12–29).

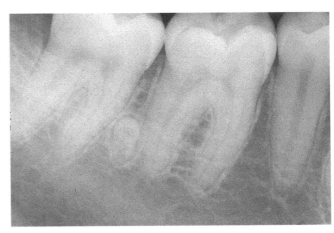

FIG. 12–29. Supernumerary tooth (or ?compound odontoma)

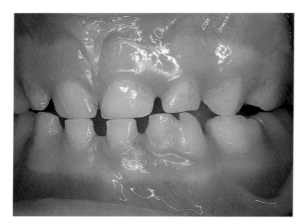

FIG. 12–30. Fusion of primary mandibular cuspid and lateral incisor

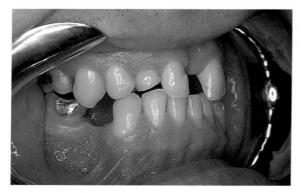

FIG. 12–31. Premolar anodontia (and transposition of cuspid)

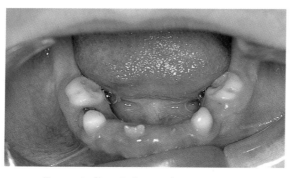

FIG. 12–32. Congenitally missing teeth

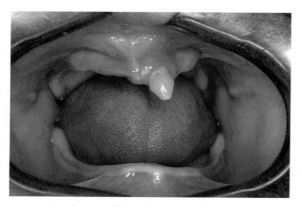

FIG. 12–33. Anodontia of hereditary ectodermal dysplasia

■ Fusion

Fusion is defined as the physical joining of two tooth germs to create a single tooth (Fig. 12–30). This may be the joining of the roots only or both the crowns and the roots. The resulting tooth is a macrodont and may be a cosmetic problem. The cause of this phenomenon is unknown.

■ Gemination

Gemination is defined as the creation or attempt to create two teeth from a single tooth germ. The result is a large tooth with two crowns and a single root, or possibly two teeth. These teeth may cause crowding and may be cosmetically unacceptable. The cause is unknown.

■ Anodontia

The failure of a tooth or teeth to develop is known as anodontia. Pseudoanodontia is a term that has been used to refer to impaction, and false anodontia to edentulism. Partial anodontia (oligodontia) is relatively common and is most likely associated with missing third molars, maxillary lateral incisors, and second premolars (Figs. 12–31 and 12–32). The cause of missing teeth is unknown. However, in *hereditary ectodermal dysplasia*, an X-linked recessive condition, affected individuals have partial or even complete anodontia (Fig. 12–33). Often only four conical-shaped teeth are seen in the canine regions. Additionally, patients with this syndrome have hypoplasia of ectodermal structures, including hair, sweat glands, and nails (Fig. 12–34).

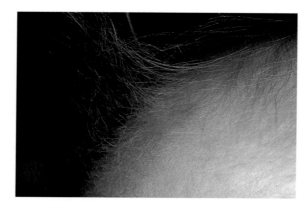

FIG. 12–34. Fine, lanugo-type hair of hereditary ectodermal dysplasia

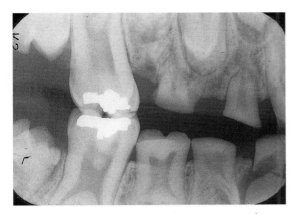

FIG. 12–35. Taurodontism (also amelogenesis imperfecta)

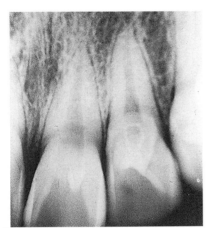

FIG. 12–36. Dens invaginatus

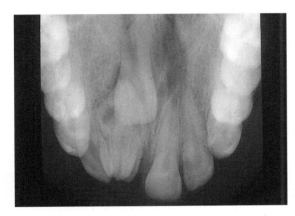

FIG. 12–37. Dens invaginatus

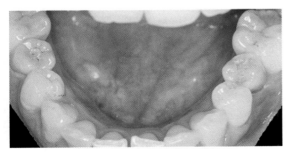

FIG. 12–38. Dens evaginatus—second premolars

■ Taurodontism

Taurodontism is an incidental finding that is defined as an elongated tooth crown or apically placed furcation giving the pulp chamber an increased size and height (Fig. 12–35). This appearance is similar to the teeth in ungulates and has been discovered in primitive populations (Neanderthals). One to all teeth may be affected. This may occur as an isolated incident, in families, or as part of a syndrome (trisomy 21, Klinefelter's). The incidence is relatively high in Inuits and people of Middle Eastern heritage. No treatment is required, and there is no significance to this curious defect.

■ Dens Invaginatus

This uncommon dental defect is also known as *dens in dente* because it appears radiographically as a tooth within a tooth (Figs. 12–36 and 12–37). It is, in fact, an exaggerated invagination of the lingual pit of usually an incisor tooth. In the extreme, the lingual pit communicates with the periapex of the tooth. The maxillary lateral incisor is most commonly affected, although it has been described in all anterior teeth, occasionally bilaterally. The cause of this defect is unknown.

The significance of dens in dente is its predisposition to early decay and pulp exposure. This is believed to be due to the patient's inability to keep the defect free of cariogenic plaque. Prophylactic filling of these defects soon after the tooth erupts is recommended. The defect can often be recognized before eruption from periapical radiographs.

■ Dens Evaginatus

This is a relatively common developmental defect that affects predominately Asians, Eskimos, and Native Americans. The defect is an accessory cusp seen in premolar teeth, often bilaterally. The accessory cusp, which is located directly in the middle of the occlusal surface, is subject to rapid wear because of occlusal abrasion (Fig. 12–38). With wear, exposure of a pulp horn in the accessory cusp occurs. This results is the appearance of a periapical lesion (periapical abscess/granuloma/cyst) in a caries-free tooth (Fig. 12–39). Because the teeth typically are young when periapical lesions develop, the pulp canals are large, making root canal therapy difficult.

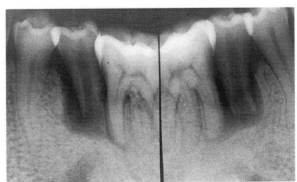

FIG. 12–39. Periapical lesions associated with dens evaginatus

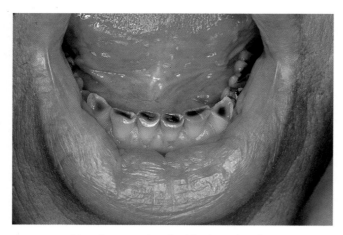

FIG. 12–40. Abrasion associated with cigar chewing

■ Attrition

Attrition is defined as physiologic wear on teeth. It is directly dependent on diet, age, and occlusal forces.

■ Abrasion

Abrasion is defined as the pathologic wearing of teeth. Abrasion occurs as the result of a habit or the use of oral abrasive substances. Among the most common etiologic agents are smokeless tobacco, pipe stems and cigars, toothbrushes, grinding, and dentifrices (Figs. 12–40 to 12–42). The location and pattern of wear is dependent on the cause and duration of use of the pathologic material. For example, common toothbrush abrasion appears as cervical notching of the posterior teeth after years of excessive brushing with a stiff-bristled brush.

■ Erosion

Erosion is the loss of tooth tissue (enamel and dentin) from the effects of acids in the mouth. The agents may be work-related (e.g., battery manufacturing) or habit-related (e.g., lemon sucking) (Fig. 12–43). Vomiting due to gastrointestinal disease or weight control in bulimia may cause erosion of the lingual surfaces of the anterior teeth. Treatment is based on identification of the cause, followed by effective counseling. Idiopathic is another category of erosion; neither habit nor occupation seems to be in effect in these mysterious cases. No satisfactory treatment is available for this group.

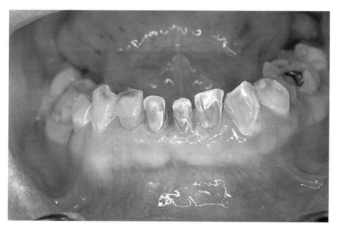

FIG. 12–41. Abrasion related to abnormal occlusal habit

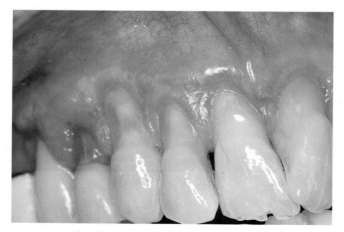

FIG. 12–42. Abrasion associated with excessive toothbrushing

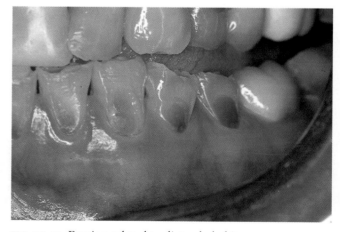

FIG. 12–43. Erosion related to diet cola habit

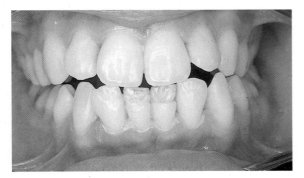

FIG. 12–44. Enamel hypoplasia, mandibular central incisors

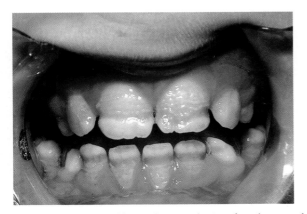

FIG. 12–45. Environmental hypoplasia: only tip of teeth normal

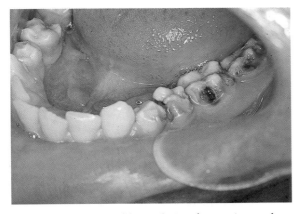

FIG. 12–46. Environmental hypoplasia of posterior teeth

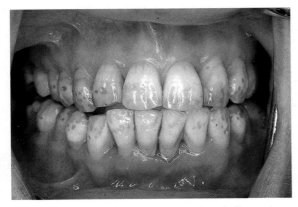

FIG. 12–47. Enamel hypoplasia associated with fluorosis

■ Environmental Enamel Hypoplasia

Interruption of enamel formation due to altered ameloblast function may be associated with environmental factors. These alterations may be of either a qualitative or a quantitative nature, and are dependent on the intensity, duration, and timing (developmental stage) of the insulting agent. These agents may affect a single tooth or an entire dentition.

Depending on severity, affected teeth can show color changes (e.g., white spots) or architectural changes (e.g., pits). The most common defect occurs in a permanent tooth crown subjacent to an abscessed or traumatized deciduous tooth (Fig. 12–44). Systemic factors, such as childhood infectious diseases, have been attributed to generalized enamel hypoplasia (Figs. 12–45 and 12–46). The physical appearance of the teeth in this instance is directly dependent on the child's age at the time of systemic disease. For permanent teeth to be affected, systemic infection must occur after birth and before age 6, when the permanent crowns are developing. If it occurs before birth, only the primary teeth and possibly the tips of the permanent incisors and first molars will be affected.

■ Fluorosis

Another etiologic factor that may cause enamel hypoplasia is toxic levels of fluoride in the diet. Greater than one part per million of fluoride in drinking water can potentially cause fluorosis. This has been associated with enamel changes ranging from white spots in mild cases to brown mottling and pitting of enamel in severe cases (Fig. 12–47).

■ Tetracycline Stain

General change in color of teeth may be associated with tetracycline ingestion during tooth development. This drug, which has an affinity for hard tissues, becomes deposited in developing teeth, imparting them with a cosmetically objectionable yellow color that oxidizes to gray with time (Fig. 12–48). This can be avoided simply by prescribing for infants one of the many alternatives to tetracycline.

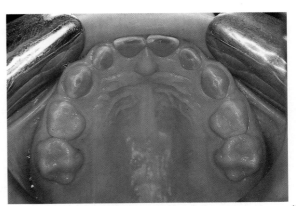

FIG. 12–48. Tetracycline stain of teeth (gray anterior, yellow posterior)

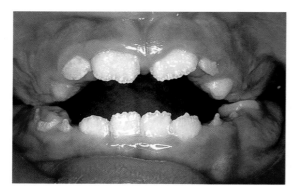

FIG. 12–49. Amelogenesis imperfecta

■ Amelogenesis Imperfecta

This is a group of similar-appearing rare hereditary disorders (autosomal dominant to recessive sex-linked) that affect the quality or quantity of both dentitions. Teeth are generally hypoplastic or hypocalcified. In the hypoplastic types, teeth erupt with insufficient amounts of enamel; in the hypocalcified types, the quantity of enamel is normal, but it is soft and friable and wears rapidly. The color of teeth in these conditions varies from opaque white to yellow or brown (Figs. 12–49 and 12–50). All teeth are affected uniformly. Radiographically, little or no enamel is detected (Fig. 12–51). The condition is of cosmetic significance, requiring full crown coverage. In spite of the soft/defective enamel, the teeth are not caries-prone.

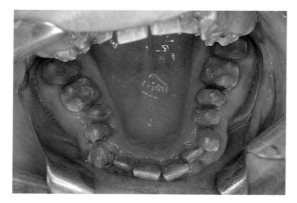

FIG. 12–50. Amelogenesis imperfecta

■ Dentinogenesis Imperfecta

This is an autosomal dominant condition that results in defective dentin of both primary and permanent dentitions. The defective dentin has a yellow translucent hue that has prompted the term "hereditary opalescent dentin." There are several subtypes described, but they share numerous clinicopathologic features. These include uniform yellow crowns with easily fractured enamel (due to poor dentin support), bell-shaped crowns, and short spiked roots (Figs. 12–52 and 12–53). In the two most commonly encountered types of dentinogenesis imperfecta (types I and II), dental pulps are replaced by opaque irregular dentin. In type III, the pulps have an unusually large profile on radiographic examination. Microscopically, dentin in dentinogenesis imperfecta has fewer and more irregular tubules.

Because of the cosmetically objectionable appearance and the extreme wear associated with this condition, full crown coverage is the treatment of choice. Although the dentin is of poor quality, crown support is usually adequate.

Dentinogenesis imperfecta may be part of a group of hereditary conditions, known as osteogenesis imperfecta, in which defective collagen is produced systemically. This is a serious systemic problem that results in extreme bone fragility and multiple fractures, hearing loss, and blue sclera (defective scleral collagen transmits melanin color of the pigmented retina).

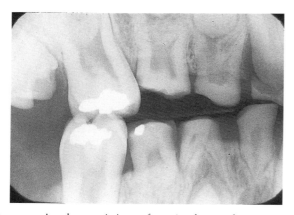

FIG. 12–51. Amelogenesis imperfecta (and taurodontism)

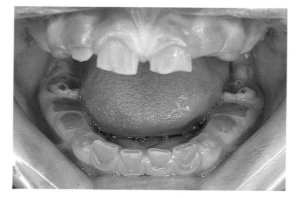

FIG. 12–52. Dentinogenesis imperfecta

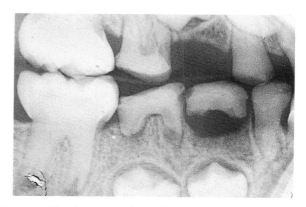

FIG. 12–53. Dentinogenesis imperfecta

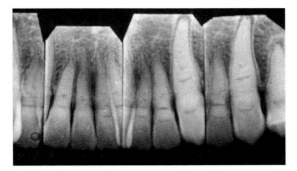

FIG. 12–54. Dentin dysplasia with bands (chevrons of residual pulp)

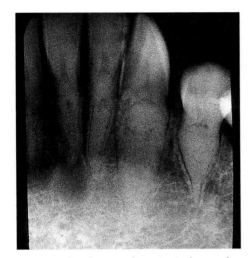

FIG. 12–55. Dentin dysplasia with periapical granuloma

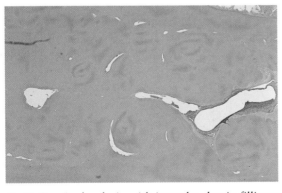

FIG. 12–56. Dentin dysplasia with irregular dentin filling pulp

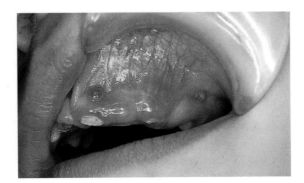

FIG. 12–57. Regional odontodysplasia

■ Dentin Dysplasia

This a rare autosomal dominant trait that affects the quality and quantity of dentin. The crowns of the teeth in this condition have a normal color and shape. Radiographically, pulps are obliterated by defective dentin and the roots are short and spiked. Thin horizontal ribbons of residual dental pulp, called chevrons, can often be seen on radiograms (Fig. 12–54). These teeth are subject to the development of periapical inflammatory disease (periapical abscess, granuloma, cyst) (Fig. 12–55). Microscopically, the pulps are filled with whorls of irregular dentin (Fig. 12–56).

A second, rarer type of dentin dysplasia (type II) has been identified. In these cases the crowns are yellow and in the permanent dentition coronal pulps, instead of being obliterated, and are remarkably large, with a profile in the shape of "thistle tubes."

Treatment is directed at retaining teeth as long as possible. However, because of the short roots and periapical lesions, the long-term outlook for saving teeth is poor.

■ Regional Odontodysplasia

The cause of this rare developmental defect is unknown. Trauma, nutritional deficiency, hereditary factors, and infection have been suggested but not well supported. This condition involves substantive deficiencies of all the hard tissues of the teeth (enamel, dentin, and cementum) in a region or quadrant of the jaw (Fig. 12–57). Tissues are thin and poorly mineralized and have been described as "ghost teeth" radiographically (Fig. 12–58). Permanent teeth are affected more than deciduous teeth, and anterior teeth more than posterior teeth. The poor quality of the affected teeth makes them of little use.

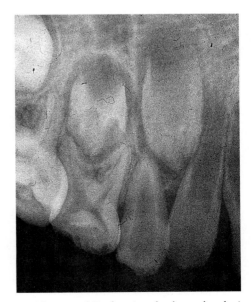

FIG. 12–58. "Ghost teeth" of regional odontodysplasia

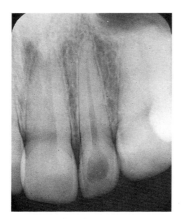

FIG. 12–59. Idiopathic internal resorption of lateral incisor

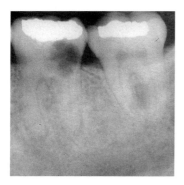

FIG. 12–60. Idiopathic internal resorption of first molar

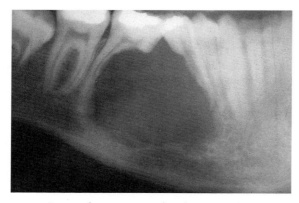

FIG. 12–61. External resorption related to central giant cell granuloma

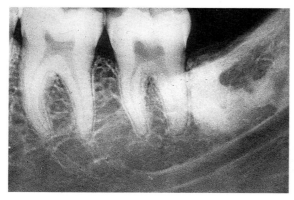

FIG. 12–62. Spontaneous resorption of impacted third molar

■ Internal Resorption

Resorption of dentin from the pulpal side may be part of pulpal inflammation or it may be idiopathic. The idiopathic form may occur in any tooth and may continue to the point of crown fracture (Figs. 12–59 and 12–60). Because of the enlarging pulp, the crown may appear pink ("pink tooth"). The treatment of choice is root canal filling.

■ External Resorption

Resorption of teeth from the external side may be due to one of several processes. Any adjacent pathologic lesion can potentially cause external resorption. This would include chronic inflammatory processes (e.g., periapical granulomas), odontogenic cysts, benign neoplasms, and malignancies (Fig. 12–61). Trauma (e.g., physical injury, excessive orthodontic force) may initiate root resorption. Impacted teeth for unknown reasons occasionally undergo spontaneous resorption (Fig. 12–62).

There is a particularly frustrating idiopathic external resorption that is virtually impossible to control, and typically leads to tooth loss. This process may affect a single tooth or the entire dentition. It appears as a gradually increasing lucency of the tooth cervix, midroot, or root apex (Fig. 12–63). Cervical and midroot resorption leads to fracture of crown from root. Apical resorption leads to tooth loss because of the increasingly unfavorable crown–root ratio. There is no detectable underlying metabolic defect, and there is no effective treatment. It has been suggested that some control may be achieved with a calcium hydroxide root canal filling (elevation of pH slows clastic process).

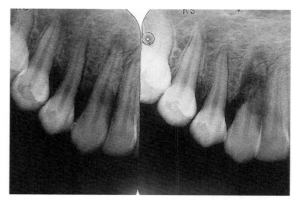

FIG. 12–63. Idiopathic external resorption (sequential radiograms)

Bibliography

CHAPTER 1 *Vesiculo-Bullous-Ulcerative Lesions*

VIRAL DISEASES

Axell T, Liedholm R. Occurrence of recurrent herpes labialis in an adult Swedish population. Acta Odontol Scand 48:119–123, 1990.

Flaitz CM, Nichols CM, Hicks MJ. Herpesviridae-associated persistent mucocutaneous ulcers in acquired immunodeficiency syndrome. Oral Surg Oral Med Oral Pathol 81:433–441, 1996.

Regezi JA, Eversole LR, Barker BF, Rick GM, Silverman S. Herpes simplex and cytomegalovirus coinfected oral ulcers in HIV-positive patients. Oral Surg Oral Med Oral Pathol 81:55–62, 1996.

BACTERIAL DISEASES

Helander SD, Rogers R. The sensitivity and specificity of direct immunofluorescence testing in disorders of mucous membranes. J Am Acad Dermatol 30:65–75, 1994.

IMMUNOLOGIC AND HEREDITARY DISEASES

Birek C, Grandhi R, McNeill K, et al. Detection of *Helicobacter pylori* in oral aphthous ulcers. J Oral Pathol Med 28:197–203, 1999.

Krause I, Rosen Y, Kaplan I, et al. Recurrent aphthous stomatitis in Behçet's disease: Clinical features and correlation with systemic disease expression and severity. J Oral Pathol Med 28: 193–196, 1999.

Marinkovich MP. The molecular genetics of basement membrane diseases. Arch Dermatol 129:1557–1565, 1993.

Porter SR, Scully C, Pedersen A. Recurrent aphthous stomatitis. Crit Rev Oral Biol Med 9:306–321, 1998.

Roujeau, JC. Stevens-Johnson syndrome and toxic epidermal necrolysis are severity variants of the same disease which differs from erythema multiforme. J Dermatol 24:726–729, 1997.

Sun A, Chang JG, Chu CT, et al. Preliminary evidence for an association of Epstein-Barr virus with pre-ulcerative oral lesions in patients with recurrent aphthous ulcers or Behçet's disease. J Oral Pathol Med 27:168–175, 1998.

Vincent SD, Lilly GE, Baker KA. Clinical, historic, and therapeutic features of cicatricial pemphigoid. Oral Surg Oral Med Oral Pathol 76:453–459, 1993.

NEOPLASMS

Bartek J, Lukas J, Bartkova J. Perspective: Defects in cell cycle control and cancer. J Pathol 187:95–99, 1999

Bryne M, Nielsen K, Koppang HS, Dabelsteen E. Reproducibility of two malignancy grading systems with reportedly prognostic value for oral cancer. J Oral Pathol Med 20:369–372, 1991.

Daley TD, Lovas JG, Peters E, Wysocki GP, McGaw TW. Salivary gland duct involvement in oral epithelial dysplasia and squamous cell carcinoma. Oral Surg Oral Med Oral Pathol 81:186–192, 1996.

Doi R, Makino T, Adachi H, Ryoke K, Ito H. Pre-operative radio-chemotherapy enhances apoptotic cell death in oral squamous cell carcinoma. J Oral Pathol Med 27:382–387, 1998.

Flaitz CM, Nichols CM, Adler-Storthz K, Hicks MJ. Intraoral squamous cell carcinoma in human immunodeficiency virus infection. Oral Surg Oral Med Oral Pathol 80:55–62, 1995.

Friedlander PL, Schantz SP, Shaha AR, Yu G, Shah JP. Squamous cell carcinoma of the tongue in young patients: a matched-pair analysis. Head Neck 20:363–368, 1998.

Hicks WL, North JH, Loree TR, et al. Surgery as a single modality therapy for squamous cell carcinoma of the oral tongue. Am J Otolaryngol 19:24–28, 1998.

Hosal AS, Unal OF, Ayhan A. Possible prognostic value of histopathologic parameters in patients with carcinoma of the tongue. Eur Arch Otorhinolaryngol 255:216–219, 1998.

Hudson DL, Speight PM, Watt FM. Altered expression of CD44 isoforms in squamous cell carcinomas and the cell lines derived from them. Int J Cancer 66:457–463, 1996.

Jones J, Sugiyama M, Speight PM, Watt FM. Restoration of alpha v beta 5 integrin expression in neoplastic keratinocytes results in increased capacity for terminal differentiation and suppression of anchorage-dependent growth. Oncogene 12:119–126, 1996.

Jones J, Watt FM, Speight PM. Changes in the expression of alpha v integrins in oral squamous cell carcinoma. J Oral Med Pathol 26:63–68, 1997.

Jordan RC, Catzavelos GC, Barrett AW, Speight PM. Differential expression of bcl-2 and bax in squamous cell carcinomas of the oral cavity. Eur J Cancer B Oral Oncol 32B:394–400, 1996.

Kropveld A, van Mansfield ADM, Nabben N, Hordijk GK, Slootweg PJ. Discordance of p53 status in matched primary tumors and metastases in head and neck squamous cell carcinoma patients. Oral Oncol, Eur J Cancer 6:388–393, 1996.

Kudo Y, Takata T, Yasui W. Reduced expression of cyclin-dependent kinase inhibitor p27 (Kip1) is an indicator of malignant behavior in oral squamous cell carcinoma. Cancer 83:2447–2455, 1998.

Kyomoto R, Kumazawa H, Toda Y, et al. Cyclin D1 gene amplification is a more potent prognostic factor than its protein over-expression in human head and neck squamous cell carcinoma. Int J Cancer 74:576–581, 1997.

Lydratt WM, Anderson PE, Bazzana T, et al. Molecular support for field cancerization in the head and neck. Cancer 82:1375–1380, 1998.

McDonald JS, Jones H, Pavelic LJ, et al. Immunohistochemical detection of the H-ras, K-ras, and N-ras oncogenes in squamous cell carcinoma of the head and neck. J Oral Pathol Med 23:342–346, 1994.

McKaig AG, Bario RS, Olshan. Human papillomavirus and head and neck cancer: epidemiology and molecular biology. Head Neck 20:250–265, 1998.

Mineta H, Borg A, Dictor M, Wahlberg P, Wennerberg J. Correlation between p53 and cyclin D1 amplification in head and neck squamous cell carcinoma. Oral Oncol 33:42–46, 1997.

Ng IOL, Lam KY, Ng M, Kwong DLW, Sham JST. Expression of P-glycoprotein, a multidrug-resistance gene product, is induced by radiotherapy in patients with oral squamous cell carcinoma. Cancer 83:851–857, 1998.

Ng Iol, Lam KY, Ng M, Regezi JA. Expression of p21/waf1 in oral squamous cell carcinomas: correlation with p53 and MOM2 genes and cellular proliferation. Oral Oncology 35:63–69, 1999.

Nisi KW, Foote RL, Bonner JA, McCaffrey TV. Adjuvant radiotherapy for squamous cell carcinoma of the tongue base: improved local-regional disease control compared with surgery alone. Int J Radiat Oncol Biol Phys 41:371–377, 1998.

Pavelic ZP, Lasmar M, Pavelic, L, et al. Absence of retinoblastoma gene product in human primary oral cavity carcinomas. Oral Oncol, Eur J Cancer 32B:347–351, 1996.

Rao DN, Shroff PD, Chattopadhyay G, Dinshaw KA. Survival analysis of 5595 head and neck cancers: results of conventional treatment in a high-risk population. Br J Cancer 77:1514–1518, 1998.

Reed AL, Califano J, Cairns P, et al. High frequency of p16 (CDKN2/MTS-1/ink4A) inactivation in head and neck squamous cell carcinoma. Cancer Res 56:3630–3633, 1996.

Riethdorf S, Friedrich RE, Ostwald C, et al. P53 gene mutations and HPV infection in primary head and neck squamous cell carcinomas do not correlate with overall survival: a long-term follow-up study. J Oral Pathol Med 26:315–321, 1997.

Schoelch ML, Le QT, Silverman S, et al. Apoptosis-associated proteins and the devolopment of oral squamous cell carcinoma. Oral Oncology 35:75–85, 1999.

Schoelch ML, Regezi JA, Dekker NP, et al. Cell cycle proteins and the development of oral squamous cell carcinoma Oral Oncology 35:333–342, 1999.

Siegelmann-Danieli N, Hanlon A, Ridge JA, et al. Oral tongue cancer in patients less than 45 years old: institutional experience and comparison with older patients. J Clin Oncol 16:745–753, 1998.

Thomas GJ, Jones J, Speight PM. Integrins and oral cancer. Oral Oncol 33:381–388, 1997.

van Oijen MGCT, Tilanus MGJ, Medema RH, Slootweg PJ. Expression of p21 (Waf1/Cip1) in head and neck cancer in relation to proliferation, differentiation, p53 status and cyclin D1 expression. J Oral Pathol Med 27:367–375, 1998.

Warnakulasuriya KAAS, Tavassoli M, Johnson NW. Relationship of p53 overexpression to other cell cycle regulatory proteins in oral squamous cell carcinoma. J Oral Pathol Med 27:376–381, 1998.

Weber RG, Scheer M, Born IA, et al. Recurrent chromosomal imbalances detected in biopsy material from oral premalignant and malignant lesions by microdissection, universal DNA amplification, and comparative genomic hybridization. Am J Pathol 153:295–303, 1998.

Yamada K, Jordan R, Mori M, Speight PM. The relationship between E-cadherin expression, clinical stage, and tumor differentiation in oral squamous cell carcinoma. Oral Dis 3:82–85, 1997.

Yamazaki H, Inoue T, Koizumi M, et al. Age as a prognostic factor for late local recurrence of early tongue cancer treated with brachytherapy. Anticancer Res 17:4709–4712, 1997.

Yuen AP, Wei WI, Wong YM, Tang KC. Elective neck dissection versus observation in the treatment of early oral tongue carcinoma. Head Neck 19:583–588, 1997.

CHAPTER 2 *White-Yellow Lesions*

REACTIVE LESIONS

Adler-Storthz K, Ficarra G, Woods KV, et al. Prevalence of Epstein-Barr virus and human papillomavirus in oral mucosa of HIV-infected patients. J Oral Pathol Med 21:164–170, 1992.

Damm DD, Curran A, White DK, Drummond JF. Leukoplakia of the maxillary vestibule—an association with Viadent? Oral Surg Oral Med Oral Pathol 87:61–66, 1999.

Eisenberg E, Krutchkoff D, Yamase H. Incidental oral hairy leukoplakia in immunocompetent persons. A report of two cases. Oral Surg Oral Med Oral Pathol 74:332–333, 1992.

Felix DH, Watret K, Wray D, Southam JC. Hairy leukoplakia in an HIV-negative, nonimmunosuppressed patient. Oral Surg Oral Med Oral Pathol 74:563–566, 1992.

Fernandez JF, Benito MAC, Lizaldez EB, Montanes MA. Oral hairy leukoplakia. Am J Dermatopathol 12:571–578, 1990.

IMMUNE DYSFUNCTION

Schifter M, Jones AM, Walker DM. Epithelial p53 gene expression and mutational analysis, combined with growth fraction assessment, in oral lichen planus. J Oral Pathol Med 27:318–324, 1998.

CHAPTER 3 *Red-Blue-Black Lesions*

RED LESIONS

Chang Y, Cesarman E, Pessin MS, et al. Identification of herpesvirus-like DNA sequences in AIDS-associated Kaposi's sarcoma. Science 266:1865–1869, 1994.

Dictor M, Rambech E, Way D, Hitte M, Bendsoe N. Human herpesvirus 8 (Kaposi's sarcoma-associated herpesvirus) DNA in Kaposi's sarcoma lesions, AIDS Kaposi's sarcoma cell lines, endothelial Kaposi's sarcoma simulators, and the skin of immunosuppressed patients. Am J Pathol 148:2009–2016, 1996.

Ensoli B, Gendelman R, Markham P, et al. Synergy between basic fibroblast growth factor and HIV-1 tat protein in induction of Kaposi's sarcoma. Nature 371:674–680, 1994.

Koehler JE, Glaser CA, Tappero JW. *Rochalimaea henselae* infection: a zoonosis with the domestic cat as reservoir. JAMA 271:531–535, 1994.

Koehler JE, Quinn FD, Berger TG, LeBoit PE, Tappero JW. Isolation of Rochalimaea species from cutaneous and osseous lesions of bacillary angiomatosis. N Engl J Med 327:1625–1631, 1992.

Miles SA. Pathogenesis of AIDS-related Kaposi's sarcoma. Evidence of a viral etiology. Hematol Oncol Clin North Am 10:1011–1021, 1996.

Morris CB, Gendelman R, Marrogi AJ, et al. Immunohistochemical detection of Bcl-2 in AIDS-associated and classical Kaposi's sarcoma. Am J Pathol 148:1055–1063, 1996.

Porter SR, DiAlberti L, Kumar N. Human herpes virus 8 (Kaposi's sarcoma herpesvirus). Oral Oncology 34:4–14, 1998.

Qu Z, Liebler JM, Powers MR, et al. Mast cells are a major source of basic fibroblast growth factor in chronic inflammation and cutaneous hemangioma. Am J Pathol 147:564–573, 1995.

PIGMENTED LESIONS

Barker B, Carpenter WM, Daniels TE, et al. Oral mucosal melanomas: the WESTOP Banff workshop proceedings. Oral Surg Oral Med Oral Pathol 83:672–679, 1997.

Batsakis JG, Suarez P, El-Naggar AK. Mucosal melanomas of the head and neck. Ann Otol Rhinol Laryngol 107:626629, 1998.

Rapini RP. Oral melanoma: diagnosis and treatment. Semin Cutan Med Surg 16:320–322, 1997.

Tanaka N, Nagai I, Hiratsuka. Oral malignant melanoma: long-term follow-up in three patients. Int J Oral Maxillofac Surg 27:111–114, 1998.

Tanaka N, Amagasa T, Iwaki H, et al. Oral malignant melanoma in Japan. Oral Surg Oral Med Oral Pathol 78:81–90, 1994.

Veraldi S, Cavicchini S, Benelli C, Gasparrini G. Laugier-Hunziker syndrome: a clinical, histopathologic, and ultrastructural study of four cases and review of the literature. J Am Acad Dermatol 25:632–636, 1991.

CHAPTER 4 *Papillary-Verrucal and Nodular Lesions*

PAPILLARY-VERRUCAL LESIONS

Gopalakrisnan R, Weghorst CM, Lehman TA, et al. Mutated and wild-type p53 expression and HPV integration in proliferative verrucous leukoplakia and oral squamous cell carcinoma. Oral Surg Oral Med Oral Pathol 83:471–477, 1997.

Palefsky JM, Silverman S, Abdel-Salaam M, Daniels TE, Greenspan JS. Association between proliferative verrucous leukoplakia and infection with human papillomavirus type 16. J Oral Pathol Med 24:193–197, 1995.

Regezi JA, Greenspan DG, Greenspan JS, Wong E, MacPhail LM. HPV-associated epithelial atypia in oral warts in HIV+ patients. J Cutan Pathol 21:217–223, 1994.

Zakrzewska JM, Lopes V, Speight PM, Hopper C. Proliferative verrucous leukoplakia: a report of ten cases. Oral Surg Oral Med Oral Pathol 82:396–401, 1996.

FIBROUS LESIONS

Desai P, Silver JG. Drug-induced gingival enlargements. J Can Dent Assoc 64:263–268, 1998.

Hajdu SI. Fibrosarcoma: a historic commentary. Cancer 82:2081–2089, 1998.

NEURAL LESIONS

Argenyi ZB, Cooper PH, Santa Cruz D. Plexiform and other unusual variants of palisaded encapsulated neuroma. J Cutan Pathol 20:34–39, 1993.

Argenyi ZB, Santa Cruz D, Bromley C. Comparative light-microscopic and immunohistochemical study of traumatic and palisaded encapsulated neuromas of the skin. Am J Dermatopathol 14:504–510, 1992.

Chauvin PJ, Wysocki GP, Daley TD, Pringle GA. Palisaded encapsulated neuroma of oral mucosa. Oral Surg Oral Med Oral Pathol 3:71–74, 1992.

Dei Tos AP, Doglioni C, Laurino L, Fletcher CDM. KP1 (CD68) expression in benign neural tumors. Further evidence of its low specificity as a histiocytic/myeloid marker. Histopathology 23:185–187, 1993.

Chrysomali E, Papanicolaou SI, Dekker NP, Regezi JA. Benign neural tumors of the oral cavity. Oral Surg Oral Med Oral Pathol 84:381–390, 1997.

Haraida S, Nerlich AG, Bise K, Wiest I, Schleicher E. Comparison of various basement membrane components in benign and malignant peripheral nerve tumors. Virchows Archiv A Pathol Anat 421:331–338, 1992.

Kaiserling E, Xiao JC, Ruck P, Horny HP. Aberrant expression of macrophage-associated antigens (CD68 and Ki-M1P) by Schwann cells in reactive and neoplastic neural tissue. Light and electron-microscopic findings. Modern Pathol 6:463–468, 1993.

Kurtin PJ, Bonin DM. Immunohistochemical demonstration of the lysosome-associated glycoprotein CD68 (KP-1) in granular cell tumors and schwannomas. Hum Pathol 25:1172–1178, 1994.

Nikkels AF, Estrada JA, Pierard-Franchimont C, Pierard GE. CD68 and factor XIIIa expressions in granular cell tumor of the skin. Dermatology 186:106–108, 1993.

Requena L, Sangueza O. Benign neoplasms with neural differentiation: a review. Am J Dermatopathol 17:75–96, 1995.

Weiss SW, Nickoloff BJ. CD-34 is expressed by a distinctive cell population in peripheral nerve, nerve sheath tumors, and related lesions. Am J Surg Pathol 17:1039–1045, 1993.

LYMPHOID LESIONS

Carbone A, Vaccher E, Barzan L, et al. Head and neck lymphomas associated with human immunodeficiency virus infection. Arch Otolaryngol Head Neck Surg 121:210–218, 1995.

Economopoulos T, Asprou N, Stathakis N, et al. Primary extranodal non-Hodgkin's lymphoma in adults: clinicopathological and survival characteristics. Leukemia Lymphoma 21:131–136, 1996.

Gaidano G, Carbone A, Dalla-Favera R. Pathogenesis of AIDS-related lymphomas. Am J Pathol 152, 623–630, 1998.

Hamilton-Dutoit SJ, Pallesen G, Franzmann MB, et al. AIDS-related lymphoma. Am J Pathol 138:149–163, 1991.

Ioachim HL, Dorsett B, Cronin W, Maya M, Wahl S. Acquired immunodeficiency syndrome-associated lymphomas: clinical, pathologic, immunologic, and viral characteristics of 111 cases. Hum Pathol 22:659–673, 1991.

Jordan RC, Speight PM. Extranodal non-Hodgkin's lymphomas of the oral cavity. Curr Top Pathol 90:125–146, 1996.

Lozada-Nur F, de Sanz S, Silverman S, Miranda C, Regezi J. Intraoral non-Hodgkin's lymphoma in seven patients with acquired immunodeficiency syndrome. Oral Surg Oral Med Oral Pathol 82:173–178, 1996.

Parker SL, Tong T, Bolden S, Wingo PA. Cancer statistics, 1997. CA Cancer J Clin 47:5–27, 1997.

Raphael M, Gentilhomme O, Tuillez M, Byron PA, Diebold J. Histopathologic features of high-grade non-Hodgkin's lymphomas in acquired immunodeficiency syndrome. Arch Pathol Lab Med 115:15–20, 1991.

Regezi JA, McMillan A, Dekker N, et al. Apoptosis-associated proteins in oral lymphomas from HIV-positive patients. Oral Surg Oral Med Oral Pathol 86:196–202, 1998.

Serraino D, Pezzotti P, Dorrucci M, et al. Cancer incidence in a cohort of human immunodeficiency virus seroconverters. Cancer 79:1004–1008, 1997.

Shapira J, Peylan-Ramun. Burkitt's lymphoma, Oral Oncology 34:15–23, 1998.

Soderholm AL, Lindqvist C, Heikinheimo K, Forssell K, Happonen RP. Non-Hodgkin's lymphomas presenting through oral symptoms. Int J Oral Maxillofac Surg 19:131–134, 1990.

OTHER CONNECTIVE TISSUE LESIONS

Falk RH, Comenzo RL, Skinner M. The systemic amyloidoses. New Engl J Med 337:898–909, 1997.

CHAPTER 5 *Salivary Gland Lesions*

IDIOPATHIC CONDITIONS

Daniels TE, Fox PC. Salivary and oral components of Sjögren's syndrome. Rheumatic Dis Clin North Am 18:571–589, 1992.

Daniels TE, Whitcher JP. Association of patterns of labial salivary gland inflammation with keratoconjunctivitis. Arthritis Rheumatism 37:869–877, 1994.

Koski H, Konttinen YT, Hietanen J, et al. Epidermal growth factor receptor in labial salivary glands in Sjögren's syndrome. J Rheumatol 24:1930–1933, 1997.

Nakamura S, Ikebe-Hiroki A, Shinokara M, et al. An association between salivary gland disease and serological abnormalities in Sjögren's syndrome. J Oral Pathol Med 26:426–430, 1997.

SALIVARY GLAND TUMORS

Batsakis JG, El-Naggar AK. Terminal duct adenocarcinomas of salivary tissues. Ann Otol Rhinol Laryngol 100:251–253, 1991.

Goode RK, Auclair PL, Ellis GL. Mucoepidermoid carcinoma of the major salivary glands. Cancer 82:1217–1224, 1998.

Milchgrub S, Gnepp DR, Vuitch F, Delgato R, Albores-Saavedra J. Hyalinizing clear cell carcinoma of salivary gland. Am J Surg Pathol 18:74–82, 1994.

Norberg LE, Burford-Mason AP, Dardick I. Cellular differentiation and morphologic heterogeneity in polymorphous low-grade adenocarcinoma. J Oral Pathol Med 20:373–379, 1991.

Norberg L, Dardick I. The need for clinical awareness of polymorphous low-grade adenocarcinoma: a review. J Otolaryngol 21:149–152, 1992.

Perez-Ordonez B, Linkov I, Huvos AG. Polymorphous low-grade adenocarcinoma of minor salivary gland: a study of 17 cases with emphasis on cell differentiation. Histopathology 32:521–529, 1998.

Regezi JA, Zarbo RJ, Stewart JCB, Courtney RM. Polymorphous low-grade adenocarcinoma of minor salivary gland: a comparative histologic and immunohistochemical study. Oral Surg Oral Med Oral Pathol 71:469–475, 1991.

Ritland F, Lubensky I, LiVolsi VA. Polymorphous low-grade adenocarcinoma of the parotid gland. Arch Pathol Lab Med 117:1261–1263, 1993.

Vincent SD, Hammond HL, Finkelstein MW. Clinical and therapeutic features of polymorphous low-grade adenocarcinoma. Oral Surg Oral Med Oral Pathol 77:41–47, 1994.

CHAPTER 6 *Cysts and Cystlike Lesions*

ODONTOGENIC CYSTS

Bataineh AB, Al Qudah MA. Treatment of mandibular odontogenic keratocysts. Oral Surg Oral Med Oral Pathol Oral Radiol Endod 86:42–47, 1998.

Crowley TE, Kaugars G, Gunsolley JC. Odontogenic keratocysts: a clinical and histologic comparison of the parakeratin and orthokeratin variants. J Oral Maxillofac Surg 50:22–26, 1992.

Garlock JA, Pringle GA, Hicks ML. The odontogenic keratocyst: a potential endodontic misdiagnosis. Oral Surg Oral Med Oral Pathol Oral Radiol Endod 85:452–456, 1998.

Honma M, Hayakawa Y, Kosugi H, Koizumi F. Localization of mRNA for inflammatory cytokines in radicular cyst tissue by *in situ* hybridization, and induction of inflammatory cytokines by human gingival fibroblasts in response to radicular cyst contents. J Oral Pathol Med 27:399–404, 1998.

Li TJ, Browne RM, Prime SS, Paterson IC, Matthews JB. p53 expression in odontogenic keratocyst epithelium. J Oral Pathol Med 25:249–255, 1996.

Nohl FSA, Gulabivala K. Odontogenic keratocyst as periradicular radiolucency in the anterior mandible: two case reports. Oral Surg Oral Med Oral Pathol Oral Radiol Endod 81:103–109, 1996.

vanHeerden WFP, Raubenheimer EJ, Turner ML. Glandular odontogenic cyst. Head Neck 14:316–320, 1992.

CHAPTER 7 *Odontogenic Tumors*

Allen CM, Hammond H, Stimson P. Central odontogenic fibroma, WHO type. Oral Surg Oral Med Oral Pathol 73:62–66, 1992.

Daley TD, Wysocki GP, Pringle GA. Relative incidence of odontogenic tumors and oral jaw cysts in a Canadian population. Oral Surg Oral Med Oral Pathol 77:276–280, 1994.

do Carmo MA, Silva EC. Argyrophilic nucleolar organizer regions (AgNORs) in ameloblastomas and adenomatoid odontogenic tumors (ACTs). J Oral Pathol Med 27:153–156, 1998.

Favia GF, DiAlberti L, Scarano A, et al. Squamous odontogenic tumor: report of two cases. Oral Oncol 33:451–453, 1997.

Funaoka K, Arisue M, Kobayashi I, Iizuka T, et al. Immunohistochemical detection of proliferating cell nuclear antigen (PCNA) in 23 cases of ameloblastoma. Eur J Cancer B Oral Oncol 32B:382–392, 1996.

Gardner DG. Central odontogenic fibroma: current concepts. J Oral Pathol Med 25:556–561, 1996.

Handlers JP, Abrams AM, Melrose RJ, Danforth R. Central odontogenic fibroma: clinicopathologic features of 19 cases and review of the literature. J Oral Maxillofac Surg 49:46–54, 1991.

Hasimoto K, Mase N, Iwai K, Shinoda K, Sairenji E. Desmoplastic fibroma of the maxillary sinus. Oral Surg Oral Med Oral Pathol 72:126–132, 1991.

Kaffe I, Naor H, Buchner A. Clinical and radiological features of odontogenic myxoma of the jaws. Dentomaxillofac Radiol 26:299–303, 1997.

Kumamoto H. Detection of apoptosis-related factors and apoptotic cells in ameloblastomas: analysis by immunohistochemistry and an in situ DNA nick end-labelling method. J Oral Pathol Med 26:419–425, 1997.

Lam KY, Chan AC, Wu PC, Chau KY, et al. Desmoplastic variant of ameloblastoma in Chinese patients. Br J Oral Maxillofac Surg 36:129–134, 1998.

Li TJ, Browne RM, Matthews JB. Expression of proliferating cell nuclear antigen (PCNA) and Ki-67 in unicystic ameloblastoma. Histopathology 26:219–228, 1995.

Li TJ, Kitano M, Arimura K, Sugihara K. Recurrence of unicystic ameloblastoma: a case report and review of the literature. Arch Pathol Lab Med 122:371–374, 1998.

Lo Muzio L, Nocini P, Pavia G, Procaccini M, Mignogna MD. Odontogenic myxoma of the jaws: a clinical, radiologic, immunohistochemical, and ultrastructural study. Oral Surg Oral Med Oral Pathol Oral Radiol Endod 82:426–433, 1996.

Maiorano E, Altini M, Favia G. Clear cell tumors of the salivary glands, jaws, and oral mucosa. Semin Diagn Pathol 14:203–212, 1997.

Mitsuyasu T, Harada H, Higuchi Y, Kimura K, et al. Immunohistochemical demonstration of bcl-2 protein in ameloblastoma. J Oral Pathol Med 26:345–348, 1997.

Mori M, Yamada T, Doi T, Ohmura H, et al. Expression of tenascin in odontogenic tumors. Eur J Cancer B Oral Oncol 31B:275–279, 1995.

Mosqueda-Taylor A, Ledesma-Montes C, Caballero-Sandoval S, et al. Odontogenic tumors in Mexico: a collaborative retrospective study of 349 cases. Oral Surg Oral Med Oral Pathol Oral Radiol Endod 84:672–675, 1997.

Myoken Y, Myoken Y, Okamoto T, Sato JD, Takada K. Immunohistochemical localization of fibroblast growth factor-1 (FGF-1) and FGF-2 in cultured human ameloblastoma epithelial cells and ameloblastoma tissues. J Oral Pathol Med 24:387–392, 1995.

Nakamura N, Higuchi Y, Tashiro H, Ohishi M. Marsupialization of cystic ameloblastoma: a clinical and histopathologic study of the growth characteristics before and after marsupialization. J Oral Maxillofac Surg 53:748–754; discussion 755–756, 1995.

Olaitan AA, Adekeye EO. Unicystic ameloblastoma of the mandible: a long-term follow-up. J Oral Maxillofac Surg 55:345–348; discussion 349–350, 1997.

Ong'uti MN, Cruchley AT, Howells GL, Williams DM. Ki-67 antigen in ameloblastomas: correlation with clinical and histological parameters in 54 cases from Kenya. Int J Oral Maxillofac Surg 26:376–379, 1997.

Roos RE, Raubenheimer EJ, van Heerden WF. Clinico-pathological study of 30 unicystic ameloblastomas. J Dent Assoc S Afr 49:559–562, 1994.

Salmassy DA, Pogrel MA. Liquid nitrogen cryosurgery and immediate bone grafting in the management of aggressive primary jaw lesions. J Oral Maxillofac Surg 53:784–790, 1995.

Schafer DR, Thompson LD, Smith BC, Wenig BM. Primary ameloblastoma of the sinonasal tract: a clinicopathologic study of 24 cases. Cancer 82:667–674, 1998.

Slootweg PJ. p53 protein and Ki-67 reactivity in epithelial odontogenic lesions. An immunohistochemical study. J Oral Pathol Med 24:393–397, 1995.

Taconis WK, Schutte H, van der Heul R. Desmoplastic fibroma of bone: a report of 18 cases. Skeletal Radiol 23:283–288, 1994.

Yamamoto K, Yoneda K, Yamamoto T, Ueta E, Osaki T. An immunohistochemical study of odontogenic mixed tumors. Eur J Cancer B Oral Oncol 31B:122–128, 1995.

CHAPTER 8 *Giant Cell Lesions of the Jaws*

Kaffe I, Ardekian L, Taicher S, Littner MM, Buchner A. Radiologic features of central giant cell granulomas of the jaws. Oral Surg Oral Med Oral Radiol Endod 81:720–726, 1996.

Lim L, Gibbins JR. Immunohistochemical and ultrastructural evidence of a modified microvasculature in the giant cell granuloma of the jaws. Oral Surg Oral Med Oral Pathol Oral Radiol Endod 79:190–198, 1995.

O'Malley M, Pogrel M, Stewart JCB, Silva RG, Regezi JA. Central giant cell granulomas of the jaws: phenotype and proliferation-associated markers. J Oral Pathol Med 26:159–163, 1997.

Pammer J, Weninger W, Hulla H, Mazal P, Horvat R. Expressions of regulatory apoptotic proteins in peripheral giant cell granulomas and lesions containing osteoclast-like giant cells. J Oral Pathol Med 27:267–271, 1998.

Whitaker SB, Waldron CA. Central giant cell lesions of the jaws. Oral Surg Oral Med Oral Pathol 75:199–208, 1993.

CHAPTER 9 *Fibro-Osseous Lesions of the Jaws*

Camilleri AE. Craniofacial dysplasia. J Laryngol Otol 105:662–666, 1991.

Slootweg PJ, Muller H. Juvenile ossifying fibroma. Report of four cases. J Craniomaxillofac Surg 18:125–129, 1990.

Slootweg PJ, Panders AK, Koopmans R, Nikkels PGJ. Juvenile ossifying fibroma. An analysis of 33 cases with emphasis on histopathological aspects. J Oral Pathol Med 23:385–388, 1994.

Souza, PEA, Paim JFO, Carvalhais JN, Gomez RS. Immunohistochemical expression of p53, MDM2, Ki-67, and PCNA in central giant cell granuloma and giant cell tumor. J Oral Pathol Med 28:54–58, 1999.

Su L, Weathers DR, Waldron CA. Distinguishing features of focal cemento-osseous dysplasia and cemento-osseous fibromas. II. Oral Surg Oral Med Oral Pathol 84:540–549, 1997.

CHAPTER 10 *Osteomyelitis*

Groot RH, van Merkesteyn JP, Bras J. Diffuse sclerosing osteomyelitis and florid osseous dysplasia. Oral Surg Oral Med Oral Pathol 82:360–361, 1996.

Koorbusch GF, Fotos P, Goll KT. Retrospective assessment of osteomyelitis. Etiology, demographics, risk factors, and management in 35 cases. Oral Surg Oral Med Oral Pathol 74:149–154, 1992.

Petrikowski CG, Pharoah MJ, Lee L, Grace MG. Radiographic differentiation of osteogenic sarcoma, osteomyelitis, and fibrous dysplasia of the jaws. Oral Surg Oral Med Oral Pathol 80:744–750, 1995.

Schneider LC, Mesa ML. Differences between florid osseous dysplasia and chronic diffuse sclerosing osteomyelitis. Oral Surg Oral Med Oral Pathol 70:308–312, 1990.

CHAPTER 11 *Malignancies of the Jaws*

Bertoni F, Bacchini P, Fabbri N, et al. Osteosarcoma: low-grade intraosseous-type osteosarcoma, histologically resembling parosteal osteosarcoma, fibrous dysplasia, and desmoplastic fibroma. Cancer 71:338–345, 1993.

Bertoni F, Dallera P, Bacchini P, Marchetti C, Campobassi A. The Istituto Rizzoli-Beretta experience with osteosarcoma of the jaws. Cancer 68:1555–1563, 1991.

Millar B, Browne R, Flood T. Juxtacortical osteosarcoma of the jaws. Br J Oral Maxillofac Surg 28:73–79, 1990.

Savera AT, Torres FX, Linden MD, et al. Primary versus metastatic pulmonary adenocarcinoma: an immunohistochemical study using villin and cytokeratins 7 and 20. Appl Immunohistochem 4:86–94, 1996.

Tanzawa H, Uchiyama S, Sato K. Statistical observation of osteosarcoma of the maxillofacial region in Japan. Oral Surg Oral Med Oral Pathol 72:444–448, 1991.

Vege D, Borges A, Aggrawal K, Balasubramaniam G, Parikh D, Bhaser B. Osteosarcoma of the craniofacial bones. J Cranio Max Fac Surg 19:90–93, 1991.

Vencio EF, Reeve CM, Unni KK, Nascimento AG. Mesenchymal chondrosarcoma of the jaw bones: clinicopathologic study of 19 cases. Cancer 82:2350–2355, 1998.

Wang NP, Zee S, Zarbo RJ, Bacchi CE, Gown AM. Coordinate expression of cytokeratins 7 and 20 defines unique subsets of carcinomas. Appl Immunohistochem 3:99–107, 1995.

CHAPTER 12 *Teeth and Periodontium*

Daley TD, Wysocki GP. Foreign body gingivitis: an iatrogenic disease? Oral Surg Oral Med Oral Pathol 69:708–712, 1990.

Furie MB, Randolph GJ. Review: chemokines and tissue injury. Am J Pathol 146:1287–1301, 1995.

Gordon SC, Daley TD. Foreign body gingivitis: identification of the foreign material by energy-dispersive x-ray microanalysis. Oral Surg Oral Med Oral Pathol 83:571–576, 1997.

Miller MD, Krangel MS. Biology and biochemistry of the chemokines: a family of chemotactic and inflammatory cytokines. Crit Rev Immunol 12:17–46, 1992.

Okada H, Murakami S. Cytokine expression in periodontal health and disease. Crit Rev Oral Biol Med 9:248–266, 1998.

Suchett-Kaye G, Morrier J-J, Barsotti O. Interactions between non-immune host cells and the immune system during periodontal disease: role of the gingival keratinocyte. Crit Rev Oral Biol Med 9:292–305, 1998.

Index

Note: Page numbers in *italics* refer to illustrations; page numbers followed by t refer to tables.